OBESITY: BEHAVIORAL APPROACHES TO DIETARY MANAGEMENT

Obesity

BEHAVIORAL APPROACHES TO DIETARY MANAGEMENT

Edited by

BEN J. WILLIAMS
Baylor College of Medicine
Department of Psychiatry

SANDER MARTIN
University of Houston
Department of Psychology

JOHN P. FOREYT
Baylor College of Medicine
Department of Medicine

BRUNNER/MAZEL, *Publishers* • New York

Copyright 1976 by Ben J. Williams, Sander Martin and John P. Foreyt

Published by
BRUNNER/MAZEL, INC.
64 University Place, New York, N. Y. 10003

Library of Congress Cataloging in Publication Data

Houston Behavior Therapy Association.
    Obesity: behavioral approaches to dietary management.

    Papers presented at the Fourth Annual Symposium of the Houston Behavior Therapy Association, Houston, Tex., co-sponsored by the Baylor College of Medicine, et al.
    Bibliography: p.
    Includes indexes.
    1. Corpulence—Psychological aspects—Congresses.   2. Behavior therapy—Congresses.   I. Williams, Ben J., 1939-   II. Martin, Sander, 1939-   III. Foreyt, John Paul.   IV. Baylor University, Waco, Tex.   College of Medicine, Houston.   V. Title.
[DNLM: 1. Obesity—Diet therapy—Congresses.
2. Behavior therapy—Congresses.   WD210 0115]
RC628.H68   1976   616.3'98'0019   75-40105

ISBN 0-87630-115-4

Foreword

A review of the behavior therapy literature in the early sixties reflects a simplistic S-R paradigm with a primary focus on systematic desensitization, aversive conditioning, modeling, and the like. Cognition, affect, sensation, perception, self-control and various social influence processes were apparently overlooked or ignored as irrelevant. And even in the mid-seventies this now largely incorrect view of behavior therapy persists in certain circles. For example, the book and popular film *Clockwork Orange* provide a typical layman's view of behavior therapy—furtive, calculating, rigid, and encouraging the docility of the robot.

Early successes within such circumscribed areas as phobias, public speaking, mental retardation, and hospitalized mental patients led to unwarranted generalization and over-zealous prediction about the potency of behavior therapy and its demonstrable ability to correct all human ills. Thus, in large measure, the naïveté and unrestrained enthusiasm of early behavior therapists produced abrasive reactions from a public at large who, on the one hand, believed these exaggerated claims and, on the other hand, feared what they felt to be an encroachment upon their personal freedom. And yet, with all this, there was an enthusiasm for the exciting gimmick and the brave new world of the emerging space age.

Today, for a variety of reasons, the situation is very different. The primary focus is now upon a self-directed, multimodal, social learning model which includes man's total internal and external environment. Guarded optimism is replacing expansive prediction.

Limitations are recognized, results reexamined and serious questions raised about ethical standards and the invasion of individual rights.

Obesity: Behavioral Approaches to Dietary Management, a highly informative and comprehensive book, is a shining example of the growth and maturation that have taken place. Williams, Martin and Foreyt, together with their associates, have succeeded in clearly demonstrating that it is possible to be rigorous and scientific without being simplistic. The scholarly and innovative studies reported here reflect not only the emerging sophistication and comprehensiveness within contemporary behavior therapy but also a vitality and overall superiority to other modes of treatment. Much as the skilled surgeon strips away pathological tissue to permit healthy cells to emerge, these authors skillfully strip away confusion and misinformation and replace it with a finished product more appropriate to our times.

This book is especially pertinent in view of the fact that obesity is one of the leading health hazards in the United States and elsewhere. Many fads and fallacies still exist regarding the etiology, maintaining variables and treatment procedures involved. Although numerous books on obesity are available, this one is unique in its combination of objectivity, rigorous evaluation and validated therapeutic innovation. The contributors, all acknowledged experts in their field, have made a resounding and lasting contribution to our understanding of both process and intervention in this important area.

DOROTHY J. SUSSKIND, Ph.D.

Professor of Educational Psychology
Hunter College of the City
University of New York

Preface

The rapid rise of learning-based therapies, including behavior modification and behavior therapy, has been unprecedented in the history of behavioral change systems. The pragmatic nature of these programs, the use of paraprofessional. and lay individuals in their administration, and the emphasis on self-help strategies have differentiated these therapies from other psychotherapies and have helped increase their popularity. Although there are many criticisms of behavior modification and behavior therapy, there is also a growing body of empirical data to attest to their effectiveness. The tools of experimental and applied behavioral analysis have been used creatively, sometimes ingeniously, with a wide range of disorders. Skinner's laboratory work on schedules of reinforcement and their subsequent application to classroom management problems, developmental disabilities, and parent-child conflicts is just one example of this phenomenon.

It was only a matter of time for the behavior modifiers to develop techniques for the treatment and control of obesity. These techniques have led to a proliferation of behaviorally-oriented weight control programs. Within the next few years, follow-up studies may indeed substantiate the use of many of these techniques as the main treatment of choice for use with obese clients. The papers in this book describe and evaluate many of these techniques now in use in this area of research.

Several important issues are emphasized in this volume. One of these is the absolute necessity for close collaboration between the behavioral therapist (be he physician, social worker, nurse, psychologist, psychiatrist, or other professional) and the nutritionist. Many behavioral therapists are ill-prepared to provide the nutrition education and diet management that represent an integral part of the total treatment program. Likewise, many nutritionists have little concept of behavioral techniques and even less experience in the instrumentation of behavioral change programs. Another related topic covered is the need for the behavioral therapist-nutritionist team to direct itself toward the family unit and diet modification as a basic change in life style. Not only must the family unit's eating behaviors change, but the affects and cognitions associated with such behaviors also may need modification, an area oftentimes neglected in weight programs. Other topics dealt with include the issue of manpower, particularly in regards to the grassroot providers of diet management, and the question of how best to provide for their adequate training and continuing supervision. National priorities as reflected in government spending, the role of advertising, and the use and regulation of the mass media are all touched on in this volume.

This book is composed of papers presented at the Fourth Annual Symposium of the Houston Behavior Therapy Association, Houston, Texas. The symposium was co-sponsored by several organizations: Baylor College of Medicine, Texas Research Institute of Mental Sciences, the University of Houston, the South Texas Dietetic Association, and the Houston Behavior Therapy Association (HBTA). Each year HBTA presents a topic of significance to behavioral therapists and others concerned with behavioral issues. We are deeply indebted to the above sponsors for their continued support of this and our other programs. We also want to thank the participants for their scholarly, thought-provoking, exciting presentations and contributions to this book. A symposium is successful only because of the hard work of many people, and at least a few hardworking HBTA members should be mentioned: Drs. Jeanne Deschner, Martha Frede, Larry Brandt, Ed Keuer, and Tom Cook. Members of the South Texas Dietetic Association, especially Ms. Barbara Kobayashi, president, Ms. Lynne Scott and Ms. Valerie Knotts, worked very hard on several aspects of the symposium. And to Ms. Susi LeBaron for her unenviable task of putting it all together into a readable manuscript, our deep thanks.

Contributors

W. STEWART AGRAS, M.D.
Department of Psychiatry and Behavioral Sciences, Stanford University School of Medicine, Stanford, California

JAMES M. FERGUSON, M.D.
Department of Psychiatry and Behavioral Sciences, Stanford University School of Medicine, Stanford, California

JOHN P. FOREYT, PH.D.
Department of Medicine, Baylor College of Medicine, Houston, Texas

ANTONIO M. GOTTO, JR., M.D., D.PHIL.
Department of Medicine, Baylor College of Medicine, Houston, Texas

CHARLES GREAVES, M.D.
Department of Psychiatry and Behavioral Sciences, Stanford University School of Medicine, Stanford, California

RICHARD L. HAGEN, PH.D.
Department of Psychology, Florida State University, Tallahassee, Florida

D. BALFOUR JEFFREY, PH.D.
Department of Psychology, Emory University, Atlanta, Georgia

VALERIE B. KNOTTS, ED.D., R.D.
Department of Nutrition and Food Science, Texas Woman's University, Houston, Texas

KATHRYN MAHONEY
Department of Psychology, The Pennsylvania State University, University Park, Pennsylvania

MICHAEL J. MAHONEY, PH.D.
Department of Psychology, The Pennsylvania State University, University Park, Pennsylvania

SANDER MARTIN, PH.D.
Department of Psychology, University of Houston, Houston, Texas

WILLIAM T. MCREYNOLDS, PH.D.
Department of Psychology, University of Missouri, Columbia, Missouri

GERARD J. MUSANTE, PH.D.
Department of Community Health Services, Duke University Medical Center, Durham, North Carolina

RONALD NATHAN, M.S.
Department of Psychology, University of Houston, Houston, Texas

BARBARA K. PAULSEN, R.D.
Lincoln University, Jefferson City, Missouri

BRANDON QUALLS, M.D.
Department of Psychiatry and Behavioral Sciences, Stanford University School of Medicine, Stanford, California

COLLEEN S. W. RAND, PH.D.
Department of Psychiatry and Behavioral Sciences, Stanford University School of Medicine, Stanford, California

JANET RUBY, A.A.
Department of Psychiatry and Behavioral Sciences, Stanford University School of Medicine, Stanford, California

LOIS SCHIAVO, M.S.
Department of Psychology, University of Houston, Houston, Texas

LYNNE W. SCOTT, M.A., R.D.
Department of Medicine, Baylor College of Medicine, Houston, Texas

ALBERT J. STUNKARD, M.D.
Department of Psychiatry and Behavioral Sciences, Stanford University School of Medicine, Stanford, California

C. BARR TAYLOR, M.D.
Department of Psychiatry and Behavioral Sciences, Stanford University School of Medicine, Stanford, California

JOHN P. VINCENT, PH.D.
Department of Psychology, University of Houston, Houston, Texas

JOELLEN WERNE, M.D.
Department of Psychiatry and Behavioral Sciences, Stanford University School of Medicine, Stanford, California

BEN J. WILLIAMS, PH.D.
Department of Psychiatry, Baylor College of Medicine, Houston, Texas

CAROLYN WRIGHT, B.S.
Department of Psychiatry and Behavioral Sciences, Stanford University School of Medicine, Stanford, California

Contents

Part I

BEHAVIORAL ISSUES

This introductory section deals with some of the outstanding issues involved in the application of behavioral techniques to weight control. In Chapter 1, "Theories of obesity: Is there any hope for order?," Dr. Richard L. Hagen examines some of the basic contradictions in the obesity literature, arguing that many different theories can account for many different types of obesity, that there are many causes of obesity, and that weight is a normally distributed variable. He stresses the need for a functional analysis not only of eating behaviors but also of exercise behaviors, and suggests that we look closer at the reinforcing value of inactivity and analyze individual differences in relation to eating sensations.

Dr. D. Balfour Jeffrey, in Chapter 2 on "Treatment outcome issues in obesity research," examines in detail a number of the parameters which prevent the effective evaluation of behavioral treatment programs and suggests possible solutions in each of the areas discussed. He examines the issue of the high attrition rate in many weight control programs, the old bugaboo called "symptom substitution," the effect of patient and therapist variables on treatment outcome, appropriate techniques for data analysis, the need for lengthy follow-ups, standardized improvement criteria, cost-effectiveness, and clinical vs. statistical significance. Jeffrey provides a strong argument for considering each of these issues when evaluating the growing number of "successful" weight control programs. Therapists need to demonstrate not only behavioral

1

changes in their clients during treatment but also self-control behaviors during extended maintenance periods, all at a reasonable cost during a reasonable time period.

In Chapter 3, "Treatment of obesity: A clinical exploration," Drs. Michael Mahoney and Kathryn Mahoney emphasize that therapists are still a long way from having any complacency in weight control regulation through behavioral means. Although behavioral techniques have generally shown better results than other techniques, the comparison does not indicate that the techniques themselves are effective. In their research article, the Mahoneys describe their multi-modal treatment program with its emphasis on training in problem solving, and provide data to support its promise as a powerful therapeutic regimen. Their study highlights the importance of cognitive factors (i.e., how people think and talk to themselves) in weight control programs and how different individuals respond to different kinds of treatments. They make a strong argument for individualizing treatment strategies for each client.

Part I provides for the reader a good summary of the state of the art, the unresolved critical issues in behavioral treatments of obesity, and the practical problems involved in running weight control research programs.

Chapter 1

Theories of Obesity: Is There Any Hope for Order?

Richard L. Hagen

As I have followed, during the past several years, the burgeoning obesity literature, I have become—like many others—more and more confused. Even this paper comes out of my typewriter with some hesitation. So many new clouds of dust have been kicked into the air that anyone who ventures into the arena with an idea is surely going to get trampled on a bit.

As Miller (1974, p. 7) reminds us, "the research shows that obese subjects do (Conrad, 1970) and don't (Abramson, 1971) exhibit psychogenic hunger. Eating does (Conrad, 1970) and doesn't (Schachter, 1971) reduce anxiety. Fat people are (Karp and Pardes, 1965) and aren't (Pliner and Kay, cited in Schachter, 1971) more field dependent than normals. The obese do (Stunkard, 1957) and don't (Stuart and Davis, 1972) risk symptom substitution as a result of dieting." In addition, the obese are (Schachter, Goldman and Gordon, 1968) and aren't (Singh, 1973) more responsive to internal cues. They do (Price and Grinker, 1973; Decke, 1971) and don't (Jackson, 1973) have a greater responsiveness to the palatability of food. And the overweight do (Cabanac, 1971) and don't (Grinker and Hirsch, 1972) defend a ponderostat weight.

Is there enough dust in your eyes? The purpose of this chapter is to wipe a few grains out by trying to impose on the plethora of views a framework which may lead us not only to better understand a seemingly confusing literature but even, perhaps, to expect it.

Where shall we begin? I suggest by agreeing with Miller (1974) and with Campbell, Hashim and Van Itallie (1971) that it is time for us to cast aside our hopes of finding a single etiological position and to recognize that we are, in all likelihood, dealing with a number of different theories which can account for different types of obesity. Furthermore, if we proceed by using a functional analysis model, exploring systematically the possible ways obesity would be expected to occur, I believe we will see a framework which fits nicely the multitude of articulated positions. The overall framework is behavioral, but it is broad enough to encompass a variety of positions. Not only might such a framework help us to understand the exasperating malady we call "obesity," it can also serve an organizational and heuristic function for many of the strategies which have been or might be employed in treatment.

In addition to the assumption of multiple etiological factors, a second very important working assumption is that all of the characteristics we shall consider are normally distributed, an assumption which is certainly in line with observations made on almost every characteristic of living organisms. To argue otherwise for a given characteristic places the onus of empirical demonstration on the one so bold to argue. Need we even point this out? Probably so. After one has read the fiftieth study involving a group of obese and a group of normals, he is tempted to adopt the belief that such discrete groups exist in the real world and then accordingly to search for discontinuous variables to account for such groups. An abandonment of the "discrete variable mentality" represents a necessary step forward in our search for reconciliation and integration of the data we now have on obesity.

Let me now briefly outline the framework we shall work with throughout this chapter. A functional analysis involves an examination of specific target behaviors, their antecedents, and their consequences. The following "ABC" framework should be a helpful memory device:

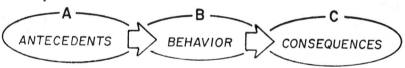

TABLE 1-1

Four possible ways in which a consequent event can affect the
frequency (probability) of a behavior which precedes it

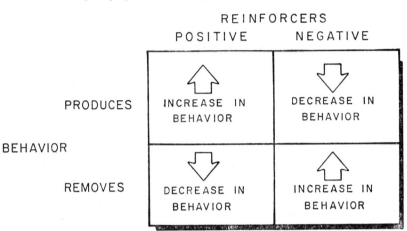

Immediately, we can see at least three main categories of events, any of which could contribute to differences in body weight. Furthermore, within these broad categories there are subcategories. Consequences, for example, can be either positive or negative in valance—or, in behavioral terms, consequences can be either positive or negative reinforcers. And, as diagrammed in Table 1-1, behaviors which have an effect on body weight can either increase or decrease depending on whether these behaviors produce or remove reinforcers. Hence, from a logical standpoint, we can expect to find a broad array of etiological factors, often leading to inconsistent research results depending upon the makeup of the particular populations studied.

BEHAVIOR

Strongly ingrained habit tells us to begin our analysis by looking at antecedents (A), but, because we find what appears to be the only point on which theorists agree under behavior (B), we will begin by looking at the middle of our framework. The point of agreement? That "obesity is . . . a consequence of a positive balance of energy consumed over energy expended" (Stuart, 1971, p. 177).

What are the behaviors (or lack thereof) which could be responsible for this energy imbalance? Two major classes of behaviors have been identified at various times by various investigators. First, there are those which bring energy into the system: those which we call . . . simply . . . "eating." And second, there are those behaviors which burn up or remove energy from the system: all behaviors which involve physical activity.

Although evidence has been garnered to indicate that the obese do not eat more than the non-obese (e.g., Johnson, Burke and Mayer, 1956; Stefanik, Heald and Mayer, 1959; Rose and Williams, 1961; McCarthy, 1966; Maxfield, 1966), such studies have dealt with obese subjects who are maintaining a steady state, and they may have little or nothing to say about food intake during that period in life when the obese individual was gaining weight more rapidly than his skinny counterpart. Under certain conditions we know that overweight people do consume more food than those of normal weight (e. g., Price and Grinker, 1973; Leon and Chamberlain, 1973). Although investigators have often done so vociferously, to deny that some people gain weight by eating more food than normals eat would involve a serious challenge to the general law of normal distribution discussed above. It is only reasonable to expect a continuum of food consumption stretching from "too much" to "too little."

What other way can people become fat? By not moving around enough to burn off excess calories. Once again, the literature is inconsistent, which is not at all surprising within an interactive model. There are indications that the obese are less active than normals (Thomas and Mayer, 1973; Glick, 1974; Johnson et al., 1956; Stefanik et al., 1959; Bullen, Reed and Mayer, 1964; Dorris and Stunkard, 1957), but differences do not always obtain (Lincoln, 1972; Bradfield, Paulos and Grossman, 1971; Huenemann, 1974).

In summary, it appears that both overeating and lack of activity contribute to obesity at various times and for various individuals. For some people, no doubt, both factors contribute. The therapist usually specifies both areas as targets, but will certainly be farther ahead if he tailors the treatment program to that set of behaviors contributing the most to his client's condition.

TABLE 1-2

Functional model for decrease in activity leading to obesity
(solid arrows) and increase in activity leading to weight
loss (segmented arrows)

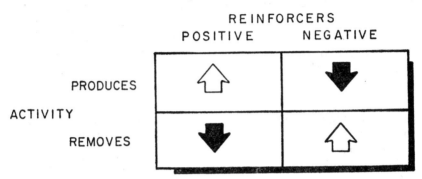

CONSEQUENT EVENTS

The frequency of a behavior will be related to those events which follow it and are contingent upon it. We can see from Table 1-2 that activity, a behavioral determinant of energy balance, can increase or decrease depending upon one of four conditions: when activity leads to (or produces) a positive reinforcer, it is likely to increase in frequency; when activity removes a positive reinforcer, it is likely to decrease. Similarly, activity will increase or decrease if it removes or produces a negative reinforcer. But why should activity level be decreased for some obese individuals? I know of no research at present which has identified "good things" removed or "bad things" produced by activity for the obese person. Thus far, researchers have concentrated on the question above: whether or not differences in activity exist. But, in the absence of research data, we may as well speculate. The first thing which comes to my mind is that activity may be reduced because activity "feels bad" or produces an unpleasant subjective experience (top right corner of the diagram in Table 1-2). Our law of normal distribution tells us that the subjective pleasure or pain associated with activity will not be the same for everyone. Furthermore, one could also speculate, of course, that activity for some people removes some of the good things in life, for example, sympathy, attention, or having someone else wait on you.

In spite of the lack of research pertaining to the question of contingent reinforcement for activity among obese and non-obese, our model can certainly serve as a guide for therapeutic intervention. Procedures for increasing energy expenditure have sometimes been questioned on the basis that the organism is likely to eat more to make up for the energy loss. What little research data we have, however, indicate that this is not true. Mayer and his colleagues have shown that under some conditions, at least, organisms will not eat enough to compensate for extra energy expended on a forced activity program (Mayer et al., 1954; Mayer and Thomas, 1967). There seems to be general agreement that we should try to increase activity in our patients, and the easiest way to do this would be to establish some positively reinforcing contingent events —praise, privileges, or a host of tangible reinforcers (top left' quadrant of Table 1-2) for such activity. But we may also want to increase activity by helping the patient establish with himself and others contracts by which increases in activity can remove aversive events (lower right-hand quadrant)—for example: "If I run three laps this afternoon, I don't have to polish the brass candlesticks tonight."

Although little is known about reinforcement of activity levels, considerably more research and theorizing have been done concerning events which seem to be responsible for increased eating. As our diagram tells us, eating will be increased when it produces "good things" or when it removes "bad things." The literature indicates that both are important.

Strongly represented for many years has been the position (Table 1-3) that eating often results in the removal of noxious emotional states ("bad things"), and is thereby reinforced (Linton, Conley, Kuechenmeister and McClusky, 1972; Leon and Chamberlain, 1973; McKenna, 1972). The immediate treatment implication is, of course, to identify the unpleasant emotional states and seek to remove them by some method which does not involve eating—for example, progressive relaxation training to eliminate tension or anxiety.

In addition to the removal of emotional distress, it has long been thought that eating is maintained because it removes or de-

TABLE 1-3
Functional model for increase of eating when
eating removes unpleasant emotional states

REINFORCERS

NEGATIVE
(UNPLEASANT STATE)

EATING

REMOVES

EATING
INCREASES

creases the aversive hunger state. Logically, one would be led to expect that the obese experience greater hunger, and consequently greater hunger reduction, than the non-obese, but experimental evidence has not borne this out. Rather, obese individuals seem to be less aware than normals of the internal states commonly referred to as "hunger," and apparently do not eat in order to decrease or remove these aversive internal states as do individuals of normal weight (Schachter, 1967). What goes on here? If the obese person does not receive reinforcement in the form of hunger reduction, wouldn't he be *less* likely rather than *more* likely to overeat?

A reasonable answer to this puzzle eluded theorists until research began to reveal that hunger has at least two parts: upper abdomen sensations and oral cravings (Jordan, 1973b). As Linton et al. (1972, p. 369) state: "for the obese, 'full' and 'not hungry' are not synonomous terms." No doubt, largely because of the dominance of positions which championed the motivational properties of drive or tension reduction (e.g., Hullian drive reduction theory; psychoanalytic theory), it simply did not occur to anyone

TABLE 1-4
Functional model for increase of eating when eating
produces pleasant gustatory experience

REINFORCERS

POSITIVE

(PLEASANT STATE)

PRODUCES	⬆ BEHAVIOR INCREASES	
EATING		

that people might eat in order to enjoy pleasure—not just to remove displeasure. The idea of eating for positive reward is now widely accepted and, as we shall see shortly, has helped us resolve the puzzle concerning why the obese individual may eat more even in the absence of hunger reduction. Indeed, the most recent addition to the theoretical perspectives is that which suggests that the obese are more highly "positively" reinforced for eating than are the non-obese; a position that leads us to focus on the upper left quadrant of our model (see Table 1-4).

The behaviorists have reminded us that many individuals spend the first half of their lives being praised by their parents for cleaning their plates and the second half being rejected by their peers for eating too much. There is no research evidence indicating that positive social reinforcement for eating occurs more often in the obese, but such might well be the case. Certainly, there is some evidence indicating that social reinforcement can effect changes in eating patterns (Stunkard and Mahoney, in press). A much more fascinating approach to the question of positive reinforcement for eating—one on which we do have an impressive amount of research—comes from theories put forth by Schachter, Nisbett and Cabanac. I find these theories particularly exciting because I came to them through the back door. Let me share my experience with you.

About five years ago, I was privileged to spend some time with Dr. Albert J. Stunkard, one of the most creative contributors to the field of obesity theory and research. At that time, Dr. Stunkard was fascinated by the accumulating evidence related to food aversions, and he had collected a large number of anecdotal reports of individuals who had developed strong food aversions by gorging themselves on a particular food. The conversation made a lasting impression on me, and when I later recounted it to a group of my students, the students challenged me to see if I could produce an experimental food aversion on myself by overeating one of my favorite foods. Not being one to easily sidestep such a "dare," the following week, while our regular research meeting was going on, I consumed about 3 good-sized boxes of chocolate-covered peanuts —a food which I had always thoroughly enjoyed. We all recognized, of course, that the unusual demands and expectations imposed on me would make my subjective impressions extremely biased data; nevertheless, we thought some ideas might be gained from the experiment.

Now, I have to admit that I no longer eat chocolate-covered peanuts even though the experience took place about 3 years ago. But the fact that I developed a dislike for the food is not what impressed me most. The first dozen bites were delicious. But by the end of the first box, the taste of the food had become very bad. By the end of the second box, the taste was really disgusting, and by the end of the third box, just the sight of the food, and the thought of eating it made me feel extremely nauseous. As I think back on this experience, I can still recreate this terrible taste in my mouth.

What did I learn that really caught my interest? First, I learned that the taste of the food progressively became worse and worse as I continued to eat. Second, I learned that what kept me from wanting peanuts in the future was the memory of that awful taste which was recreated in my phenomenal sensory experience each time I looked at or thought about the food. The first of these

Palatability of a given food as a function of the amount of that food
consumed (theoretical relationship)

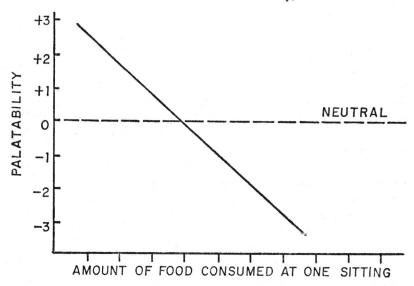

experiences shoved me in a certain direction theoretically, and the
second has led me into some interesting treatment experiments.

After the food-gorging experience, I assumed that if I had
plotted the "palatability" of the food against amount consumed,
I would have gotten a function somewhat like that in Figure 1-1.
Under normal circumstances, I suppose I would have stopped
eating before, or certainly by the time, the palatability of the food
approached a neutral rating, suggesting, what to me at the time,
was a new way of thinking about satiety. Then it occurred to me
that, assuming a normal distribution of slopes, the amount of food
consumed before reaching a neutral point would differ across
people, leading some to be skinny, some to be normal, and some to
be fat. It can be seen, for example, in Figure 1-2 that individuals
with a flatter slope would consume far more food before reaching
a neutral point than would those whose satiety slope is steep.

Hence, the following week at my research group, we all gorged
ourselves. While keeping ratings of palatability, we each ate about

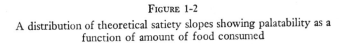

FIGURE 1-2

A distribution of theoretical satiety slopes showing palatability as a function of amount of food consumed

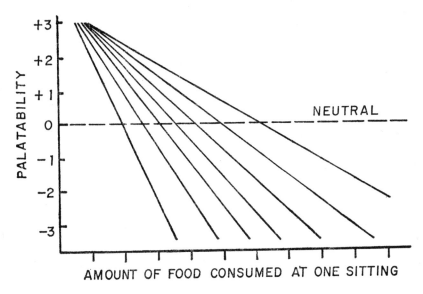

15 average-sized pieces of fudge. Many variables were uncontrolled, but we figured that as a pilot study the project would give us enough information to decide in which direction to go next. I had not told any of the students what my hunches were, but, true to prediction, the skinny members showed a very rapid decline in palatability while the two fat members of the group showed almost no decline at all. We discussed the data, and one of my students became interested enough to research the literature in preparation for a master's project. What we found, of course, many of you already know. Precisely the same sort of study had been carried out by Cabanac and Duclaux (1970) and by Cabanac, Duclaux and Spector (1971). These investigators had found that obese subjects continued to rate a sucrose solution as pleasant even after stomach loads of glucose solutions. Non-obese subjects, on the other hand, reported a post-ingestion decrease in rated pleasantness for the sucrose solution. Another series of experiments (Wooley and Wooley, 1974) indicate that a caloric ingestion

sufficient to inhibit salivation (appetite?) in non-obese does not do so in the obese—additional support for the position that slopes of change in gustatory experience may be different for obese and non-obese.

My student, David Gilbert, tried to replicate Cabanac's results, but he did not find that obese and normal weight subjects differed in the slopes of their palatability ratings. Instead, he found that the absolute ratings of pleasantness differed significantly (Gilbert, 1973), with the obese subjects rating the sucrose solutions as more pleasant both before and after ingestion of the solution. A number of procedural differences could have led to these differing results, the most important of which appears to be that Gilbert's subjects were moderately obese while Cabanac's subjects were considerably obese. We should remember, however, that just as we should expect "satiety slopes" to be normally distributed, leading some people to eat more than others before they are satiated, so also we should expect the absolute amount of pleasure received from eating to be normally distributed, leading some people to eat more because the absolute "distance" to the neutral point would be greater. Either condition could contribute as a cause of obesity.

Evidence for the hypothesis that the gustatory experience of the obese individual is often more pleasant than that of his thin counterpart comes also from several other studies. Linton, Conley, Kuechenmeister and McClusky (1972) found that when subjects were asked to rate pictures of a variety of foods, obese subjects more often rated the foods as pleasant and appealing. Wooley, Tennenbaum and Wooley (unpublished) observed meal choices by 2,732 individuals in cafeterias representing distinctly different levels of palatability and found that the obese were significantly over-represented at the good cafeteria and under-represented at the bad one. These results are certainly consonant with the finding by Goldman, Jaffa and Schachter (1968) that obese college students were more likely to cancel dormitory food contracts in order to eat in better restaurants and with the data reported by Schiffman (1973) indicating that obese subjects were better able to identify foods by taste alone (other cues removed) than were normal weight subjects. After reviewing the studies in this area, Wooley and Wooley (unpublished) conclude that the obese do, indeed, appear to be somewhat hyper-responsive to palatability, but only at high levels of palatability—that is, when the food is very good. Furthermore, they conclude that the single factor which has most consistently differentiated the responses of obese and normal subjects has been that of palatability.

It has also been suggested by Nisbett (1972) and by Cabanac and Duclaux (1970), who elaborated Schachter's theory, that the subjective pleasantness of food (and its change during ingestion) is affected by whether one is under, at, or above a biologically determined "set-point" weight. According to this position, the subjective pleasantness of food will be different for people who are under their biological "set-point" than for those who are at or over it.

Support for this position is sketchy but certainly merits our attention. Cabanac, Duclaux and Spector (1971), in what must be considered more a pilot study than anything else, themselves went on a weight reduction diet, losing between 8 and 10 percent of their body weights. They took the pre- and post-ingestion taste tests (referred to earlier in this chapter) just as their subjects had in earlier experiments. Before the diet, all three reported a change in the taste of the sucrose solution from pleasant to unpleasant after the ingestion of a glucose solution, but after dieting they reported that the taste of the sucrose solution no longer decreased in pleasantness after glucose ingestion. These results are consonant with those reported by Nisbett, Hanson, Harris and Stair (1973), who found that rats which were maintained on a negative energy balance showed increased acceptance of good tasting food and increased rejection of bad tasting food. From a review of other pertinent literature, Jordan (1973a, page 20) concludes: "Quite clearly, then, the organism resists alterations in energy balance in either direction and defends its body weight." Research now strongly indicates that the defense lines are drawn primarily by changes in the subjective pleasantness of food—that is, the under-weight organism eats more because the food tastes better (or tastes better for a longer period of time), while for the stabilized organism food intake is reduced because of the lower reward value of food. If this hunch is correct, one would expect obese subjects who have been staying somewhat below their "set-point" because of social pressures, limited wardrobe, or what-have-you, to behave in regard to food somewhat differently from stabilized obese subjects and normal weight subjects (Nisbett, 1972; Cabanac and Duclaux, 1970). It would seem reasonable to assume, for example, that subjects who volunteer for weight reduction programs are less stabilized than obese subjects who are sought out by investigators. Discouragingly, there really is no good way to discriminate between stabilized and non-stabilized individuals, but certainly recent investigations suggest that the experimenter should at least make some attempt at discrimination. The vast majority of studies have not made any efforts to determine the status of their subjects' weight stabilization, thus opening the door to an additional source of confusion in the literature.

Maybe I am biased because of my own introduction to the area with the chocolate-covered peanuts, but the literature I've read so far leads me to predict that more and more attention will be given to differences between obese and non-obese on the dimension of "how much food is liked," both in absolute terms and over periods of ingestion. I have always been one to test theory first by asking whether or not my grandmother would have believed it. In this case, I think she would have—even though she wasn't obese. I have no doubt that many obese people would also tell us we are on the right track. In fact, they've been telling us this for years, but we haven't been listening. Anyone who has worked for any length of time with weight problems has heard the following comments time and again: "Oh, how I would just love to have a chocolate sundae!" "Why, Doc, I can eat a whole box of candy at one sitting . . . I just crave the stuff."

What do these comments tell us? If we take them at face value, they mean that the person trying to lose weight has "in his mind's mouth" the dream of a taste which will bring him indescribable pleasure, a dream which seldom, if ever, occurs in the mind of a skinny individual.

The problem with this view, of course, is that it lacks esoteric sophistication. What journal editor is going to get excited about a paper which says that fat people eat too much because they like food better than skinny people do? That's precisely what his grandmother would have told him, too. The position may be doomed to obscurity simply because it is too close to what everyone believes.

Nevertheless, the theory does have important implications for treatment, some of which have been put into practice for years. If obese individuals do eat more because their gustatory experience is more positive, a good practice would involve taking the edge off the appetite, or providing gustatory satisfaction with low caloric foods (many programs recommend this procedure).

Secondly, the above hypothesis points toward the use of food aversion techniques. Although electric shock as an aversive UCS was among the first aversion techniques used (Meyer and Crisp, 1964; Thorpe, Schmidt, Brown and Castell, 1964), recent applications of aversion procedures have concentrated on the use of noxious odors paired with the highly palatable foods (Kennedy and Foreyt, 1968; Foreyt and Kennedy, 1971) and the use of covert sensitization, a technique developed by Cautela (1966).

Still another implication from the "gustatory pleasure" theory of overeating is that, for a highly suggestible subject, hypnosis might be effective in changing the subjective pleasure associated with eating. In addition, a technique which thus far has not appeared in the literature may also have some promise. Conceivably, one could overeat a particular food far beyond the "point of neutral taste" until the subjective experience created by the sight, smell, or taste of the food is highly aversive. It seems reasonable to assume that people approach and consume food because their memory of the last time they tasted it tells them that the experience would be pleasant. Few of us are going to choose foods we remember as having tasted bad. Would it be possible to have an individual eat a specific food so far beyond the point of neutral taste (see Figure 1-2) that there would be implanted in his memory a very strong aversive image which would be elicited by the sight or smell of the food? The theory of satiety suggested earlier in this paper suggests that it would be possible.

ANTECEDENT EVENTS

There remains now one category of events in our functional analysis framework which has not been discussed: events which are antecedent to those behaviors which result in a positive energy balance. Behaviorists call these antecedent events discriminative stimuli, or stimuli, which signal the occasion upon which a behavior is likely to be reinforced. When eating takes place in the presence of certain stimuli and is accordingly reinforced—by pleasant gustatory experiences, for example— the stimuli become discriminative for eating. These stimuli, or cues, may be conveniently categorized as "internal" and "external."

Eating to Internal Cues

A decade ago, Stunkard and Koch (1964) demonstrated that obese subjects were not as capable as normals of recognizing sensations arising from the gut, sensations which are often referred to as "hunger." Since that time, a number of studies (Schachter, 1967, 1968, 1971) have led Schachter and his colleagues to take the position that, whereas the normal subject often eats in response to internal states of hunger, "the eating behavior of the obese is relatively unrelated to any internal gut state" (Schachter, 1968, p. 136). Coming from a psychosomatic approach, Bruch's (1973) position is very similar. Bruch holds also that the obese do not correctly identify internal states of hunger, but instead eat in response to a variety of unpleasant physical or emotional states. If true, one would certainly expect eating to take place more often in the obese simply because there is a greater frequency of internal states which signal eating. McKenna (1972) has provided some data which lend support for this position.

Eating to External Cues

It has also been proposed that, for the obese, eating is controlled to a greater degree by external cues, such as sight of food and the time of day. An impressive array of studies has provided evidence for this position (e.g., Nisbett, 1968; Schachter and Gross, 1968; Goldman, Jaffa and Schachter, 1968; Stutz, Warm and Woods, 1974). Furthermore, an elaboration of this basic proposition has included the claim that external cues per se do not count; rather, it is the salience of the cues which is important (Pliner, 1973, 1974). Wooley and Wooley (unpublished) point out that none of the "external cue" literature is totally convincing and that many contradictory studies have appeared; nevertheless, my feeling is that enough evidence exists to make a fairly strong case for greater external cue control for at least some segments of the obese population.

Suppose some people do eat to external cues and some to internal hunger cues. Why should one group eat more than the other? The argument is the same we presented earlier for the "undifferentiated internal state" theory of Bruch (1973). The more states or conditions there are which come to exert control over eating, the more the person is likely to eat. And from a logical standpoint, there exists a greater variety of possible external cues than internal ones.

One of the earliest behavioral treatment strategies (Ferster, Nurnberger and Levitt, 1962) emphasized the elimination of those external cues which seem to exert discriminative control over eating. The person, for example, who eats because of the sight of food is asked to eliminate extraneous foods from around the house, or to at least keep them shut away in the cupboard where they cannot be seen. Research evidence over the past decade does seem to provide an empirical base for such discriminative control strategies.

SUMMARY AND OVERVIEW

What have we suggested? First, that there are probably many reasons people are overweight. The single theory simply will not do any longer. Second, from a logical standpoint, each of the multitude of factors which could lead to a positive balance of energy is probably normally distributed, leading to the prediction that the probability of finding data supporting the etiological significance of such factors is quite high, depending upon what population one studies. Third, I have suggested that the behaviorist's functional analysis approach provides us with a framework into which we can integrate the major theories on the market today. This framework not only tells us that people eat, and overeat, for a variety of reasons, but also relates logically to a variety of procedures—most already in use—which can help these individuals regulate their food intake.

Chapter 2

Treatment Outcome Issues in Obesity Research

D. Balfour Jeffrey

Obesity is a complex phenomena which we are just beginning to understand and treat effectively. Numerous behavior modification studies indicate that these principles and procedures offer a promising treatment for obesity (Abramson, 1973; Hall and Hall, 1974; Stunkard and Mahoney, in press). However, to fully evaluate the effectiveness of behavior treatments or any treatment for obesity, a number of issues in therapy outcome research need to be considered. The purpose of this chapter is to examine some of these treatment outcome issues in obesity research.

Attrition

People dropping out prematurely from traditional treatments for obesity has frequently been a major problem, and recent studies indicate it is no less a problem for learning-based therapies (e.g., Harris and Bruner, 1971). In research studies, subjects can be lost either equally or unequally across the different interventions, and either during treatment or follow-up. In all cases, the higher the attrition rate, the more difficult it is to interpret the results. For example, in the Harris and Bruner study (1971) on weight reduction, the contingency contract subjects who stayed

Portions of this paper are drawn from Jeffrey (1974a and 1975a).

in treatment did better than the self-control subjects; however, the contract group had a 58% dropout rate while the self-control group had no dropouts. If the dropouts were included in the contract group, then the self-control group would have performed better.

Romanczyk et al. (1973) conducted an interesting comparative analysis of various behavioral techniques in the treatment of obesity. In general, their results indicated that all of the self-management procedures were more effective than a no-treatment control or self-monitoring for weight. The authors concluded that the sustained weight losses suggested that the subjects learned behavioral skills which they were able to implement on a continuing basis. Hopefully, this interpretation is correct. However, these researchers, as all researchers, have the same problem of analyzing and interpreting follow-up data when there are high dropout rates (over 30% at posttreatment and over 60% at follow-up for the Romanczyk et al., 1973 study). A plausible rival hypothesis is that the "sustained" weight loss was simply due to the fact that 17 of 28 patients who dropped out between pretreatment and follow-up had not lost weight or even gained weight. If data from the dropouts had been included in the analysis, perhaps the posttreatment and follow-up data might not have been so impressive. The problem of attrition occurs frequently and is difficult to handle in obesity outcome research. However, if this issue is not resolved it can seriously jeopardize the validity of a study.

One solution is to continue to collect data on the dropout subjects and to include them in the data analysis (Harris and Hallbauer, 1973). If it is impossible to include dropouts in the analyses, then subjects for which there is incomplete data might be excluded entirely from the statistical analyses (Jeffrey, 1974b). The best solution is to minimize dropouts. One promising procedure for minimizing dropouts is a deposit contract contingent on completion of the program (Hagen, Foreyt, and Durham, 1976). In addressing themselves to the problem of follow-up attrition, Sobell and Sobell (1973) recognize that conducting a follow-up takes time and persistence; however, they make recommendations which, if instituted, should increase the return rate. These include: (1) tell the subjects from the beginning of the program the details and purpose of the follow-up, (2) make the follow-up frequent and personal, and (3) obtain the names of friends and relatives of the subject who will probably have contact with him during the follow-up. Thus, collateral sources of information are available to assess the reliability of the subject's report and to provide information in case the subject is not available.

Symptom Substitution

The issue of "symptom substitution" has divided psychodynamic and behavior therapists about treating the "symptoms" rather than the "underlying cause" (Ullmann and Krasner, 1965). Traditional psychodynamic approaches are based on personality systems in which the symptom is seen as the expression of deep underlying psychological conflicts. It is assumed that if the symptom is eliminated without treating the "underlying cause," the formation of a new sympton will occur.

The newer behavior therapy approaches consider symptoms as behaviors which are acquired and maintained by learning principles just as any other behavior is acquired and maintained. It is assumed that the maladaptive behavior (symptom) is a function of environmental discriminative and reinforcing stimuli; consequently symptom substitution is not expected to occur if the maladaptive behavior is treated with learning principles.

The issue is further obfuscated by extreme positions, i.e., symptom substitution always occurs (Bookbinder, 1962) or it never occurs (Yates, 1958) in behavior therapy. Bandura (1969) argues that symptom substitution is an important psychological issue but little will be made in resolving this issue if it continues to be misconstrued as one of non-symptomatic versus symptomatic treatment. Bandura concludes that all forms of psychotherapy affect behavior changes through either deliberate or unwitting manipulations of controlling variables. Both psychodynamic and behavior therapists are equally concerned with modifying the "underlying" factors of maladaptive behaviors. However, these theories differ in what they consider the "causes" of the maladaptive behavior.

In discussing the symptom substitution issue, Cahoon (1968) argues that symptom substitution (a maladaptive behavior) can occur within any therapeutic approach and whether it actually occurs is an empirical rather than a theoretical matter. For example, the treatment of obesity with hypnosis often leads to short-term effects lasting only a few days; the treatment of obesity with only contingency contracting (Mann, 1972) leads to undesirable side effects such as patients resorting to the use of diuretics, steam baths, and vomiting to meet weight loss goals; the treatment of obesity with "diet pills" has proven to produce only transitory weight losses and to have adverse side effects (Rivlin, 1975).

Since symptom substitution or adverse side effects may occur with any therapeutic technique, it is important to collect these kinds of data. An excellent example of an empirical approach to this problem is in the experimental treatment of obesity by Wollersheim (1970). She found that behavior modification was the most successful treatment, that there was a reduction in anxiety among her successful subjects, and that there were no indications of symptom substitution. Harris (1969) also found no evidence that behavioral treatments for weight loss resulted in emotional disturbance or symptom substitution.

In a review of traditional therapy and dieting treatments for weight reduction, Stunkard and Rush (1974) found an increase in depression and emotional illness in the obese as they lost weight. The behavioral approaches generally have found little evidence of symptom substitution. However, since so much is still unknown about obesity, Stuart (1973) has recommended that behavioral researchers continue to monitor for symptom substitution. In fact, it would be prudent for all researchers to continue to collect data on the possibilities of symptom substitution or side effects so that this question can be continually answered by empirical facts rather than by theoretical fiat.

Patient and Therapist Variables

The results produced by a new treatment often mask the fact that even in successful studies there are great individual differences in patient improvement. In surveying the traditional psychotherapy outcome research, Bergin (1971) found that treated patients performed more variably on the post-measures than untreated patients. He also found that some patients in "successful" treatment groups did not improve and some even got worse. Similar findings appear in the obesity literature (e.g., Harris and Bruner, 1971; Penick et al., 1971).

The frequency and level of variability could be ascertained if researchers report individual subject data in addition to group data, or at a minimum report the standard deviation of weight losses, note if there are "unsuccessful patients" in a "successful treatment," and make available upon request the individual data. Possible sources of this response variation include techniques that vary in effectiveness, and patients and therapists who vary in their ability to implement behavioral techniques.

Traditional psychotherapy research has stressed patient and therapist variables, sometimes to the extent of ignoring treatment variables (Bergin and Garfield, 1971). However, the emphasis in behavior therapy research has been just the opposite. The initial emphasis on learning principles was needed in the early stages of behavior therapy, but it is now time to also include relevant patient and therapist variables into the domain of behavioral research. Paul (1969), for example, recommends including the relatively stable personal-social characteristics and physical-life-environmental characteristics of both the patient and therapist as appropriate domains of behavior modification inquiries. Research suggests that important variables are the expectancy and interpersonal skill of the therapist, and the motivation, expectancy, and social economic status of the patient (Fiske et al., 1970; Bergin and Garfield, 1971).

Although most behavioral obesity studies allude to patient and therapist characteristics, the primary emphasis is on learning-based treatment procedures. In some of these studies (e.g., Martin and Sachs, 1973; Stuart, 1967) a plausible rival hypothesis for the outcome of these studies is that the patient's motivation and expectancy, as well as the therapist's interpersonal skill and expectancy, rather than the learning principles, accounted for positive results. In the final analysis the issue of therapist and patient variables can best be answered empirically by the inclusion of these variables in obesity research. Furthermore, it would be useful for some investigations to conduct factorial experiments which evaluate the effects of treatment, patient, and therapist variables, as exemplified in the Wollersheim (1970) study on obesity.

Data Analyses

In presenting descriptive statistics of different weight treatments, investigators do not present the same statistics. For example, some studies report mean weight loss, while others report median weight loss. Some studies report standard deviations or ranges of different treatments, while others do not report any measure of variability. It would be helpful in interpreting the results if studies at least presented the number of subjects, mean weights, range, and standard deviation for each group across pretreatment, posttreatment, and follow-up.

In the common pretest-posttest group design, the statistical procedure typically used for analyzing therapy outcome is to calculate a gain (or difference) score for each subject and then to determine with a *t* test or simple analysis of variance if there is a significant difference between the control group and experimental group. However, both Harris (1963) and Cronbach and Furby (1970) argue that, because of regression effects and errors of measurement, tests performed on raw gain scores are inadequate. Instead, they recommend either an analysis or variance with blocking or an analysis of covariance. Feldt (1958) and Elashoff (1956) provide statistical guidelines for when either blocking or an analysis of covariance should be used. If the correlation between the covariate (e.g., the pretest score) and the variate (dependent variable) is greater than .6, Feldt (1958) recommends that the analysis of covariance be used as it provides the greatest precision or power (assuming of course the other assumptions for the analysis are fulfilled). For example, in obesity research, the correlation between preweight and postweight is generally about .8; consequently, it is preferable to use an analysis of covariance to test for differences across groups (Jeffrey, 1974b; Jeffrey and Christensen, 1975). If the correlation between the covariate is between .4 and .6, then an analysis of variance with blocking is recommended. Analysis of covariance and blocking analysis of variance have generally not been conducted; however, with their clear statistical advantages and the advent of electronic computers for high speed calculations, these statistical tests are recommended for assessing differences between groups.

Follow-up

Generalization across time involves the maintenance of the desired behavior after the treatment phase has ended. Obviously, the first phase of an obesity treatment program must demonstrate some change in the primary dependent variable—a reduction in weight—before the issue of maintenance becomes important. Numerous studies now show that behavioral procedures have produced significant weight losses (Abramson, 1973; Jeffrey, in press; Stunkard and Mahoney, in press).

An equally important issue is whether the treatment changes are maintained. The initial enthusiasm in drug and psychodynamic therapies for the treatment of obesity has proven to be ill-founded when long-term, empirically based follow-ups have been conducted (Stunkard and McLaren-Hume, 1959). Much of the recent enthusiasm for behavior modification approaches has been based on dramatic demonstrations of weight loss over short periods of time. However, two recent behavior studies (Hall, 1972; Hall et al., 1974) have not found maintenance of weight over extended follow-ups, while other behavioral studies have shown promising long-term follow-ups (Harris and Hallbauer, 1973; Stuart, 1967). The history of research on obesity indicates there is still insufficient long-term, follow-up data to go beyond guarded optimism about the efficacy of behavior therapy in the treatment of obesity. There is now a clear need to include 6 month, 1 year, and longer follow-up in weight investigations so as to determine the durability of the behavioral changes. Such empirically derived data may temper our enthusiasm about a particular program, but it may also provide a better basis for modifying and improving treatment procedures. The editorial policy of *Journal of Behavior Therapy and Experimental Psychiatry* and *Addictive Behaviors* to require follow-up data of at least 6 months is a good incentive for researchers to begin to routinely collect and report long-term data.

Standardized Improvement Criteria

In obesity research, standardized improvement criteria need to be established so that studies can be meaningfully compared. For example, it is difficult to compare directly a study that reports a behavior-therapy group losing an average of 13 pounds (Wollersheim, 1970) with a study that reports 53% of the patients in a behavior-therapy group losing more than 20 pounds (Penick et al., 1971).

Feinstein (1959), in an article on the measurement of success in weight reduction, discusses the advantage of various indices such as pounds lost and percentage of subjects who lost weight. He concluded with a recommendation for a new index called the weight-reduction index (RI), which is equal to the percent of excess weight loss $\times$ relative initial obesity. This index takes into account weight, height, amount overweight, goal, and pounds lost.

$$RI = [(W_1/W_s) \quad (W_1/W_t)] \ 100$$

Where:

W_1 = weight loss; W_s = surplus weight
W_1 = initial weight; W_t = target weight

The reduction index will usually provide a value between 0 (no weight loss) and 200 (a large weight loss). For example, if a subject initially weighed 250 pounds, had a target weight of 150, had a surplus weight of 100 pounds, and lost 50 pounds, then his weight-reduction index would be

$$\frac{50}{100} \times \frac{250}{150} \times 100 = 83.$$

If he had lost 100 pounds, his weight-reduction index would have been 166, and if he had failed to lose any weight, his RI would be 0.

The advantage of developing a standardized index for reporting weight loss is the convenience it offers in comparing the effectiveness of different weight-reduction treatments, regardless of theoretical orientation and procedures. In the interim between the development and acceptance of standardized improvement criteria, it would seem valuable to report, or at least to make available upon request, the results for every subject so that sufficient data will be available for later comparisons.

Cost-Effectiveness

Patterson, Ray, and Shaw (1968) wrote, "It seems important for social engineers not only to assess the relative permanence of their efforts, but also to provide data describing the amounts of time required as an investment to produce these effects" (p. 54). There is a clear mandate to develop interventions which not only have effects and persist but which also are feasible in terms of cost.

There are presently no clear guidelines on how to proceed in assessing cost factors. Some of the factors that might be considered include: (1) there should be a regular tabular reporting of the number of contacts, therapist's time, amount of money spent for therapist-client interactions, and client's work on his own, as suggested by Patterson (1969), Jeffrey and Christensen (1975) and Stuart (1967); (2) the social cost of the maladaptive behaviors of the patient needs to be more adequately assessed (e.g., the cost in terms of increased health problems and medical expense might be assessed for normal weight and overweight); and (3) a comprehensive decision-making model for evaluating the cost of inappropriate behaviors versus the cost of implementing alternative treatment programs might be utilized. In this way, more rational, humane decisions can be made about which treatment programs to implement (Arthur, 1969; Davidson, Clark, and Hamerlynck, 1974).

If obesity treatment studies reported how much time was spent per session and total time with each patient, an efficiency measure could be calculated. One cost-effectiveness index might be the mean weight-reduction index divided by the mean treatment time per patient (Jeffrey, 1975b).

$$\text{Cost-Effectiveness Index} = \frac{\text{Mean weight-reduction index}}{\text{Mean treatment time per patient}}$$

Clinical Significance

Basic and analogue research are necessary to understand the mechanisms of obesity and to isolate the different components of a treatment program. Statistical procedures are often used to determine whether the findings were significant. For example, Manno and Marston (1972) report that both positive covert reinforcement and negative covert sensitization were statistically more effective than a minimal treatment control group in producing weight losses. Even though the two behavioral treatments were statistically significant, most people would probably agree that the reported

4- or 5-pound weight loss during treatment would be clinically insignificant. It is not always easy to determine criteria for clinical significance. However, most obese patients and health professionals involved with the treatment of obesity would probably say that a patient needs to achieve a substantial part of his weight goal and maintain that weight loss for a least 6 months to a year before they would consider the finding clinically significant.

There are now ample studies which show behavioral treatments to be statistically superior to traditional treatments for obesity (Hall and Hall, 1974; Stunkard and Mahoney, in press). The question which now needs to be answered is whether behavioral treatments are clinically significant. This is an empirical question which future research will need to answer.

Summary

The goal of most treatments for obesity is to help the patient so that he can learn to manage his own weight. Unfortunately, the enthusiasm for new approaches for treating obesity often are not thoroughly evaluated to see if in fact they are really helping people to reduce and maintain their weight loss. A number of treatment outcome issues—attrition, symptom substitution, patient and therapist variables, data analyses, follow-ups, standardized improvement criteria, cost-effectiveness, and clinical significance—have been discussed which should be considered in evaluating any treatment program for obesity. Hopefully, researchers and clinicians alike will consider these treatment outcome issues in conducting and evaluating obesity treament programs.

Chapter 3

Treatment of Obesity: A Clinical Exploration

Michael J. Mahoney and
Kathryn Mahoney

Although the behavioral treatment of obesity has harvested results which are refreshingly more optimistic than those of more traditional methods, the need for further research and clinical refinement is substantial (Stunkard and Mahoney, in press). As has been pointed out elsewhere (Mahoney, 1975a), the fact that behavioral strategies are more effective than others does not imply that they are therefore very effective. We remain a long way away from any semblance of justification for complacency in weight regulation. Significant poundage losses are still in the minority and long-term maintenance has remained seldom examined.

In evaluating the power of a therapy procedure, one must consider factors other than the magnitude and permanence of change. For example, the consistency of the procedure is a very important consideration for the counselor. Although behavioral strategies are consistently superior to other treatment methods, they are often very inconsistent across subjects. Individuals receiving the same treatments often vary tremendously in their responsiveness. One person may lose forty pounds, several others will shed from ten to thirty, and one or two will show no change or even a slight weight gain.

What are the factors which account for these variations? A number of researchers have searched unsuccessfully through such variables as locus of control, hereditary patterns, age, childhood versus adult-onset obesity, and so on. With a small handful of exceptions—such as the observation that males are more successful than females—none of the suspected variables have been successful predictors. Extensive analyses of psychometric and questionnaire data have likewise been unsuccessful.

An alternative method for identifying predictor variables might be to *intensely* study a small number of individuals in the hopes of finding clinically suggestive clues regarding their differential responsiveness. With that goal in mind, the present project was begun.

METHOD

The subjects were 13 adult volunteers (9 female, 4 male) who had been screened for contraindicative variables (colitis, regional ileitis, etc.). Participants were required to leave a $20 deposit, which was returned to them contingent upon attendance ($10 at 12 weeks; $10 at one year). The treatment program was preceded by a two week baseline period. During the ten subsequent weeks, group meetings were conducted. In each weekly session, technical information was imparted, homework assignments were given, and participants received feedback and individual assistance on prior assignments and specific problems. Four therapists participated.* Technical information and self-regulatory training was divided into eight major categories.

1. *Self-Monitoring.* Subjects recorded their daily eating habits in three categories (quantity, quality, and situational control). Emphasis was placed on *behavior change* rather than *weight loss* (Mahoney, 1974a). Actual food intake was also recorded for three days during baseline and again after six weeks of treatment. These data were subsequently used to evaluate the nutritional adequacy of the program (Welles, 1973).

2. *Nutritional Counseling.* Participants were instructed in the basic principles of digestion and food metabolism. Emphasis was placed on the importance of a reasonable and well-balanced diet which could be integrated into a permanent lifestyle.

3. *Physical Activity.* Subjects were encouraged to develop in-

---

* The authors thank Bill Fernan and Fran Mason for their invaluable assistance.

dividualized and reasonable methods for increasing their energy expenditure. Emphasis was placed on expanding daily activity patterns rather than initiating strenuous calisthenic exercise. Attention was given to the beneficial effects of physicial activity on hunger, fat mobilization, maintenance, and cardiovascular functioning.

4. *Stimulus Control.* Subjects were informed of the role of physical stimuli in eating behavior (Ferster, Nurnberger, and Levitt, 1962; Stuart, 1967, 1971). Five homework assignments were employed: (a) separating eating from other activities, (b) making high calorie foods unavailable or inconspicuous, (c) altering the size and appearance of food portions, (d) eating slowly, and (e) the reducing of eating to avoid waste.

5. *Relaxation Training.* After an explanation of its relevance for emotional eating, participants were given tape recorded instructions and homework assignments designed to teach them muscular relaxation skills.

6. *Social Support Engineering.* Subjects were instructed in methods of developing adequate social support for their continuing reduction efforts. The families of participants were invited to all sessions, one of which was devoted to their role in the program. They were asked to (a) restrict their feedback to praise (no teasing or criticism), (b) avoid offering the subject food (either at or between meals), and (c) cooperate by compromising their own meal and snack patterns in a way which was beneficial to the subject. The subject, in turn, was instructed to shape and socially reinforce the reinforcer (e.g., spouse), thereby generating a reciprocally helpful pattern.

7. *Self-Reinforcement.* Participants were asked to draw up individualized self-reward contracts which specified reasonable goals and incentives. To insure consistent follow-through, contracts were witnessed, signed, and monitored by family members or friends.

8. *Cognitive Ecology.* Because of the critical role of cognitive symbolic processes in self-regulation (Thoresen and Mahoney, 1974; Mahoney, 1974b), participants were taught to "clean up what they said to themselves." This was effected by their being trained in the recording, evaluation, and alteration of weight-

relevant private monologues. Treatment emphasis was placed on their standard setting and self-reactions.

After completion of the formal 10 week treatment program, subjects underwent a follow-up procedure which was designed to wean them from formal structured counseling in a gradual fashion. For the first year, follow-up contacts were scheduled at increasing intervals (2, 3, 4, 5, 6, 6, 7, and 7 weeks). During the second year, contacts occurred approximately every three months.

Results and Discussion

Program and follow-up data are summarized in Table 3-1. Twelve subjects completed the ten week program. After a relatively consistent increase during baseline, the average post-treatment loss was 9.0 pounds.* At six months this had increased to almost 18 pounds, where it stabilized for the remainder of the two years.

Inspection of Table 3-1 suggests several tentative conclusions regarding the present study. First, as anticipated, subjects displayed considerable variability in their responsiveness to the program. There were a few "star" losers in the 20-50 pound range, some others losing very little, and the rest in between. Maintenance was a particularly difficult problem. Many of our group had lost substantial poundage by the six-month follow-up. If we had stopped there, our study would have looked relatively impressive in both magnitude and consistency. However, at subsequent follow-up contacts there was considerable relapse on the part of three subjects. At the two-year contact, the individual losses ranged from less than a pound to over 46 pounds (standard deviation = 16.5). Three subjects were particularly successful. The males did substantially better than the females and there was a tendency for less successful subjects to terminate earlier. Both of these findings have important implications for the conduct of research and reporting of results in obesity treatment. Similarly, the data suggest the possibility that "seasonal" parameters may require attention in future inquiries. There was a slight tendency for participants to lose weight during the warmer months and to regain it, or at least

---

* As noted in the table, poundage lost is calculated from *pre-baseline* weight, thereby yielding a more conservative index of loss in most instances.

TABLE 3-1
Program and Follow-Up Data

Subject	Sex	Age	Height	Pre-Weight	Skinfold[a]	Baseline	Treatment	6 mo.	Weight Loss[b] 1 year	18 mo.	2 years	Skinfold Change 1 year	Family Support[d]
1	F	61	63.0	172.5	22.3	1.0	12.5	17.5	9.0	3.5	0.5	6.0	1.00
2	F	44	65.5	164.9	21.0	0.0	10.5	16.0	13.0	12.0	10.5	5.5	2.50
3	F	36	62.5	173.5	23.7	+11.0	2.0	5.0	7.5	9.5	31.0e	7.9	3.0
4	F	36	64.5	173.0	21.7	0.0	8.0	10.0e	—	—	—	—	2.75
5	F	27	65.5	156.0	16.7	+5.0	3.0	7.5	—	—	—	—	1.50
6	F	29	62.5	204.5	19.7	+4.0	2.5	—	—	—	—	—	2.00
7	F	29	69.0	189.0	19.3	+3.5	10.5	27.7	—	—	—	—	3.00
8	F	30	64.5	168.5	20.0	+1.0	—	—	—	—	—	—	1.50
9	F	53	60.0	149.0	16.3	+2.0	+1.5	—	—	—	—	—	2.50
Mean		38.3	64.1	172.2	20.1	+2.8	5.9	13.9	9.8	8.3	14.0	6.5	2.19
10	M	38	71.5	293.0	26.3	3.0	22.5	30.5	28.5	29.0	24.0e		3.00
11	M	29	68.0	196.0	19.0	0.5	16.5	30.5	48.5	48.0	46.5e		2.75
12	M	58	65.5	205.0	19.0	+3.0	2.0	14.5	5.0	—	9.0e	1.7	1.75
13	M	27	70.0	225.5	20.0	2.5	19.5	19.0	8.5	—	5.5e	3.3	2.75
Mean		38.0		229.1	21.1	0.8	15.1	23.6	22.6	—	21.2	—	2.56
Total (pooled)						+1.7	9.0	17.8	17.1	20.4	18.1	4.9	2.31

a. Averaged skinfold thickness (in mm.) of chin, cheek, and right triceps.
b. Balance beam measurement; recorded losses are relative to pre-baseline weight.
c. Note that this subject *gained* 11 pounds during baseline; her total in-program loss was 42 pounds.
d. Average support as independently rated by four therapists during week 10 (1 = poor, 3 = good).
e. Self-reported by mail.
— Dropped.

show less progress, during Fall and Winter. This trend, if substantiated by more controlled research, would have important bearing on the external validity of brief studies which are initiated in colder seasons and terminated in the summer.

A second major finding was the apparent relationship between participants' success and an index of the social support. During the tenth week of the program, each subject was given a social support score based upon family attendance and their reports regarding the cooperation and encouragement they received from family and friends. These independent ratings by each of the four therapists were then averaged for a summary score. Using weight loss in pounds as the covariate, the correlation between treatment outcome and social support was .92 at the end of the ten-week program ($p < .01$, n $= 12$). It dropped to .33 at six months (n $= 10$) and .39 after one year (n $= 7$). It should be noted however, that four of the least successful subjects terminated during this interval. The removal of their variance from the correlation may therefore partially account for the reduction. This possibility is further suggested by inspecting the 18-month and two-year correlations. The former was .51 (n $= 5$), with two of the least successful remaining subjects absent from the weigh-in. At two years their weights were obtained by mail and the final correlation between reduction and social support was .63 (n $= 5$). These data are, of course, only suggestive, but the relatively high correlations obtained with such a small sample are noteworthy.

Evaluations of the nutritional adequacy of the program were undertaken to see if weight losses produced by behavioral strategies were obtained at the cost of sound nutrition. A nutritionist scored baseline and treatment phase records of food consumed (type and quantity). Each participant was rated on the adequacy of his intake of specified vitamins, minerals, and proteins (as determined by Federally recommended standards). These were converted to the Mean Daily Adequacy Ratio, a recognized index of nutritional status. Within-subject comparisons showed no deterioration in nutritional adequacy from baseline to treatment ($t = 1.20$, n. s.). Moreover, comparisons with participants in two local chapters of national self-help groups showed the behavioral participants to be generally equivalent and occasionally superior to these samples (Welles, 1973).

At their first follow-up contact, subjects were asked to fill out a questionnaire regarding the possible transfer of their new skills to other areas of personal functioning. Ninety percent reported that their relaxation training had generalized beneficially to such diverse areas as test anxiety, fear of flying, traffic jams, and insomnia. Similarly, seventy percent said that their cognitive skills had helped them in handling other personal problems (e.g., finance management, compulsive housecleaning, and academic performance). Throughout the two years of the program there were no reported instances of deleterious treatment effects (i.e., "symptom substitution").

Two other findings of the program are somewhat more difficult to convey since they lack quantification. In our opinion, however, this does not negate their potential clinical significance. In the numerous interviews conducted with program participants, two phenomena were apparent to all four therapists: (a) the importance of cognitive variables, and (b) marked individual differences in subjects' "favorite" techniques. As outlined elsewhere, perfectionistic standards, negative beliefs, and self-defeating private monologues were common obstacles to success (Mahoney and Mahoney, 1975). Early in our program we had introduced an assignment on cognitive ecology—"cleaning up what you say to yourself." This was basically designed to train participants in the detection and alteration of such maladaptive thought patterns as the following:

"This will never work—I always regain whatever I lose."

"It is so unfair that some people can eat all they want without gaining weight."

"I think I'm just naturally fat."

"You can't expect me to diet when I have a cold."

We pointed out that monologues like these are a very effective way to sabotage one's reduction efforts. Another way is to set perfectionistic standards.

"I'm never going to binge again."

"After tonight, no more desserts until I've lost 20 pounds."

"I'm going to avoid all bread and starches."

Each of the above is, of course, almost impossible. Because they demand all-or-none criteria for feeling good about yourself, they often lead to "saint versus sinner" psychology. As soon as you violate the perfection goal—with your first heavy meal, or donut, or piece of garlic bread—you figure, "The hell with it, I just blew my diet!" This philosophy leads to a repetitive cycle of aborted diets, perhaps two or three a year, in a yo-yo pattern which nutritionist Jean Mayer (1968) calls the "rhythm method of girth control."

Although we were reasonably confident that cognitive ecology would be helpful to our participants, we had no idea *how* important it would be. Judging from their comments and our own clinical observations, the cognitive components of our program may well have been the most important (Mahoney and Mahoney, 1975).

A third finding in our study had to do with individual differences in responsiveness to the remaining elements in the program. Some participants, for example, found stimulus control strategies to be very helpful. Others reported that these techniques were not at all beneficial. For them, relaxation training may have been a key strategy. Still others liked our physical exercise suggestions or self-reward contracts. This tremendous variability across participants suggested two lines of research to us.

First, it suggested that many of the popular assumptions in the treatment of obesity may warrant re-examination. For example, it is often taken for granted that overweight clients are overeaters and that they exhibit something called "the obese eating style." This is characterized by rapid eating, relatively few (but large) bites, and a hypersensitivity to food-related cues. We have now completed five studies examining these clinical assumptions (Gaul, Craighead, and Mahoney, 1975; Mahoney, 1975a, 1975b). Their results have been generally non-supportive. We found, for example, that obese individuals may not be faster eaters than normal weight persons. They do not seem to take fewer bites, and there is some recent evidence that they may not be hypersensitive to external stimuli (Wooley and Wooley, 1975).

The validity and clinical impact of this research on the obese eating style cannot, of course, be evaluated at this stage of the data. One implication, however, is very clear—we have been too long remiss in examining our basic assumptions in the treatment of obesity. If our preliminary findings hold up under replication and methodological refinement, they suggest that obesity cannot be accurately portrayed as a product of one universal behavior pattern. Like the elusive traits of personality psychology, the obese eating style may turn out to be one of those Barnum phenomena with very limited clinical relevance. Weight problems may be complexly individualized in their development, maintenance, and treatment. For one person, inadequate physical activity may be a primary factor. Another may overeat due to nervous tension or boredom. A third may be obsessed with food thoughts to the extent that they dominate—and exacerbate—weight loss efforts. Judging from our experience, most instances of obesity seem to derive from a combination of influences—and the combinations seem to vary from one individual to the next.

This individual variability lent impetus to our reappraising the relatively fixed format of our treatment package. It suggested the possible benefits of structuring future programs to allow personalization of strategies. By training the individual in applied problem solving skills, we anticipated that they would be able to tailor their reduction efforts to their own personal needs. We also felt that such skills would be helpful as general coping strategies for long-term maintenance (Mahoney, 1974b). The counselor can seldom dedicate the rest of his life to assisting one group of weight watchers. At some point in time they must be weaned of professional assistance and left to their own self-improvement skills. We now feel that problem solving training may be a critical element in optimal counseling and have revised our weight control program accordingly (Mahoney and Mahoney, in press). Judging from the available literature and our own problem solving probes during the two-year follow-up of our study, it may well be one of the most powerful therapeutic elements we can provide.

CONCLUSION

The foregoing data, of course, are far from demonstrative. As reflected in the goals and methodology of the program, our efforts were intentionally exploratory rather than experimental. Heuristics are but one of the valuable aspects of intensive clinical research. The extreme variability in subject responsiveness, for example, stimulated a series of studies which have re-examined some of the common assumptions in the behavioral treatment of obesity

(Mahoney, 1975a, 1975b; Gaul, Craighead, and Mahoney, 1975). Moreover, our clinical explorations suggested the need for major revisions in our treatment program along the lines of increased emphasis on social support, cognitive skills, and the personalization of strategies (Mahoney and Mahoney, in press). Forthcoming evaluations of these revisions will hopefully further refine our expanding knowledge and efficacy in this area.

Part II

BEHAVIORAL TECHNIQUES

Many of the issues discussed in Part I are dealt with in this Part II. In Chapter 4, "Stimulus control as the behavioral basis of weight loss procedures," Dr. William T. McReynolds and Barbara Paulsen review the A B C paradigm and support the position that the key to behavioral control of eating lies in the *A* portion of the paradigm, that stimulus control of behavior is the answer to weight loss and maintenance. Their paper is in strong agreement with that of Hagen's. Both deal with the failure of the "stop mechanism" to operate in the obese and conclude, therefore, that the key to weight loss is in the control of the antecedent conditions leading to eating behaviors. McReynolds and Paulsen describe their program at the University of Missouri and Lincoln University involving a behavioral therapist-nutritionist team and present 18-month follow-up data supporting the efficacy of their program in both weight loss and, more importantly, weight maintenance. Their results suggest that behavioral treatments emphasizing the elimination or reduction of eating cues in an obese person's environment can have significant and lasting effects. They also argue convincingly for the use of behavioral therapist-nutritionist treatment teams.

In Chapter 5, "Effect of deposit contracts and distractibility on weight loss and maintenance," Dr. John P. Vincent, Lois Schiavo, and Ronald Nathan demonstrate the use of behavior modification strategies emphasizing the *C* of the A B C paradigm, i.e., deposit

41

contracts. Particularly interesting in this article is their detailed discussion of the practical problems involved in this type of research.

Chapter 6, "A proposal for a macro environmental analysis in the prevention and treatment of obesity," by Dr. D. Balfour Jeffrey, spans the entire A B C paradigm and may be viewed as a social development paper encompassing social learning and operant developmental theories. Jeffrey describes how society shapes behavior, including the stimuli presented in our environment as we grow up (i.e., the A), the contingency management of our behavior by those around us (e.g., our parents insisting we clean our plates, TV advertising, availability of junk foods with little warning to parents that these foods have little nutritional value, etc. (i. e., the C), and the difficulty in changing our behavior (i.e., the B) without any basic changes in either A or C. Jeffrey focuses not on the analysis of eating, exercise, and the psychological patterns of the individual, but on our whole society, discussing how society oftentimes impedes the development of good eating or exercise habits. He shows how society, through its various social, governmental, and educational components, along with the public media, serves to reinforce overeating and poor dietary habits. He cites, for example, the effect that Saturday morning advertisements on children's television programs have on the consumption of sugar-coated cereals, many of which contain more than 50% sugar. Among Jeffrey's proposals for increasing the good eating habits of our society are the need for improved nutrition education, better food labeling, and changes in the use of vending machines and in the advertising of specific foods, and a reassessment of the role of subsidies and taxes on food buying and food consumption. He also suggests proposals for improving the physical education habits of our society, including better physical education programs, establishment of national standards for sports and recreational facilities, increased emphasis on employer-sponsored sports facilities, and an examination of the relationship between our tax structure and physical activity.

Part II gives the reader an opportunity to look at the specific behavioral techniques being used in weight control programs and presents some stimulating ideas on improving the overall health of our society.

Chapter 4

Stimulus Control as the Behavioral Basis of Weight Loss Procedures

William T. McReynolds and
Barbara K. Paulsen

The day will come when a behavior modifier writing for a general professional audience will not have to begin with an explanation of what behavior therapy or behavior modification* is. Today is not such a day. Confusion as to the exact nature and characteristics of behavior therapy or "behavior mod" is widespread in the public mind. Indeed, agreement among recognized *authorities* on the matter has been relatively scarce until recent years. Early descriptions of behavior therapy provided by Eysenck (1959, 1970; Eysenck and Rachman, 1965) and Wolpe (1969), for example, identify the application of "modern learning theory" and learning paradigms to human behavioral problems as characteristic features. Definitions offered first by Ullmann and Krasner (1965) and Skinner (1956, 1966), in contrast, emphasize a focus on overt, observable behavior as well as the use of the principles and procedures of learning. Each of these broad conceptions of behavior therapy has brought forth fundamentally different criticisms and defenses of the field as a whole (Breger and McGaugh, 1965; Eysenck, 1971; Locke, 1971; Portes, 1971; Rachman and Eysenck, 1966; Waters and McCallum, 1973; Wiest, 1967).

---

* The terms behavior therapy and behavior modification are used interchangeably within this chapter reflecting the absence of an accepted convention governing their differential use.

More recently, such influential contemporary thinkers as Albert Bandura (1969), Leonard Krasner (1971), Frederick Kanfer and Jeanne Phillips (1970), Gordon Paul (1969), Todd Risley (1969), and Aubrey Yates (1970) have popularized a characterization of behavior therapy as a fundamentally empirical, scientific approach to understanding and changing unwanted behavior. Within this broad point of view there are two subtly different perspectives. The first emphasizes a reliance on empirically grounded behavior principles to achieve wanted behavior changes:

> The unifying factor in behavior therapy is its basis in derivation from experimentally established procedures and principles. The specific experimentation varies widely but has in common all the attributes of scientific investigation including control of variables, presentation of data, replicability, and a probabilistic view of behavior. (Krasner, 1971, pp. 487-488)

In a phrase, this view of behavior therapy identifies it as an applied branch of experimental psychology.

The second, still empirically oriented perspective on behavior therapy, highlights the independent investigative nature of applied behavioral activities. Thus,

> Behavior modification is experimental research investigating variables which alter significant human behaviors—behaviors not selected for their convenience or relevance to theory, but precisely because they have been identified by society as being important to man—not pale analogues to important behaviors, but those behaviors themselves. Behavior modification is therapy: the alterations produced in the important behaviors are required to be therapeutic—they must be improvements of sufficient magnitude to actually benefit the client, his family, and society. (Risley, 1969, p. 103)

Behavior therapy, then, is an experimental branch of applied (clinical, social, and educational) psychology.

Common to both these fundamental contemporary viewpoints on the nature of behavior therapy is their concern with the processes of knowing in applied treatment endeavors and belief in the preeminence of scientific methodology in the development of procedures for the control of human behavior. Important in their interface is the complementary nature of the views of the behavior therapist as *both* a scientist-therapist and a behavior change technologist.

The development of the now numerous behavior therapies has tended to conform logically to the conceptual sentiments expressed by Krasner (1971) and others, although there have been a few notable adherents to the alternative, applied research approach (Lazarus and Davison, 1971; London, 1972). The derivation of the treatment procedures from basic research following the "experimental psychology applied" view has resulted in a predominant reliance on the processes known (i.e., empirically supported) to govern learning or conditioning and the performance of learned responses. Operant and respondent conditioning and modeling procedures were the first point of departure or derivation from basic research. Thence we were given the characterization of behavior therapy as the application of "modern learning therapy" by Eysenck, Rachman, Wolpe and others. Learning "theory" was a good place to start, and practically everyone did begin there in earlier days. But the animal or learning lab imposes no necessary or definite limits on this expansive area. Today there is growing and impressive evidence (e.g., D'Zurilla and Goldfried, 1971) of behavior therapy's broad base as both an applied branch of experimental psychology and an experimental branch of applied psychology. Research on the behavioral treatment of obesity contributes much in this regard.

BEHAVIOR THERAPY FOR WEIGHT CONTROL

An audience of American professionals needs little documentation of the prevalence and seriousness of obesity in this country. The many and familiar estimates of the number of obese people in the United States vary around the figure of 50 million, or 25 percent of the total population. Until recently, however, the status of professional treatment and control of obesity was that "most obese patients will not remain in treatment. Of those who do remain in treatment, most will not lose significant poundage; and of those who do lose weight, most will regain it promptly" (Stunkard, 1958, p. 87). Taking these "mosts" to be a conservative

51 percent we find that 87 percent of the people treated for obesity receive no or only temporary relief.

The problem is not that people are unconcerned about their bulging waistlines. Indeed, a poll conducted in 1964 (reported in Wyden, 1965) revealed that upwards of 25 million Americans were, at that time, either actively dieting or "watching" their weights. The sale of appetite depressants alone has been reported to reach a high of $80,000,000 (Fee, Wilson and Wilson, 1969). The unflattering reality of the situation has been that psychologists, nutritionists, and physicians have had little to offer the overweight individual seeking an effective and practical way of losing and keeping off unwanted pounds.

The application of behavior modification techniques to the problem of weight control appears to be changing this dismal picture. Three broad behavioral approaches, all of which have been derived largely from research on the acquisition and performance of learned responses, have been investigated. The first, aversion procedures, has made use of primary and covert aversive stimulation within a respondent conditioning paradigm. In these procedures, food thoughts (e.g., imagining the sight of a preferred food) or actual food stimuli (e.g., food odors) are paired with aversive odors or thoughts of nausea in an effort to reduce the palatability of food via a conditioned aversion response. Foreyt and Kennedy (1971), in one of the few even partially controlled studies of aversive procedures, compared the effects of the repeated pairing of favored foods and noxious odors with the results of the popular Take-Off-Pounds-Sensibly (TOPS) program. The authors give no description of their version of the latter program, and even though the aversion therapy resulted in significantly greater weight losses (a mean of 13.33 lbs. versus 1.0 lbs. after nine weeks of treatment), it is unclear just to what it is superior. Two recent and more conclusive studies by Janda and Rimm (1972) and Manno and Marston (1972) compared covert sensitization (Cautela, 1967) with untreated or contact only groups. The covert aversion procedure, entailing the pairing of mental images of food and eating with feelings of nausea and vomiting, produced comparatively small but stable weight losses in the magnitude of 10 lbs. with 4-6 weeks of treatment.

A second behavior therapeutic approach to weight loss utilizes operant reinforcement-punishment procedures. Case studies by Ayllon (1963), Bernard (1968), and Moore and Crum (1969) have all demonstrated the feasibility of promoting rather large weight losses through the use of favorable or unfavorable consequences contingent on changes in weight or eating habits. Harmatz and Lapuc (1969) found significantly greater reductions among patients receiving money contingent on weight losses than among patients receiving "social pressure" group therapy and diet only. Similarly, contractual reinforcement wherein subjects turn over sums of money or valuables which are then returned in small amounts contingent on weight loss has proven superior to no treatment (Jeffrey and Christensen, 1972; Mahoney, 1974), monitoring without reinforcement (Mahoney, 1974; Mahoney, Moura and Wade, 1973; Mann, 1972), information only (Mahoney et al., 1973), and information plus encouragement (Jeffrey and Christensen, 1972). Weight loss *rates* associated with this treatment have been a respectable 1-3 pounds off per week, although total amounts of weight taken off often have been only 6-8 pounds.

The most widely studied and consistently effective behavior control procedure for weight loss was first suggested by Ferster, Nurnberger and Levitt (1962) in their classic analysis of the control of eating. This treatment is a collection of behavioral, self-control techniques which aim at teaching obese people how to achieve control of their eating by understanding and manipulating the antecedent and consequent conditions of that behavior. Supplemented in recent years but basically unchanged, the therapeutic potpourri includes training in stimulus control, self-reinforcement and punishment, controlled deprivation, response chaining, self-monitoring, response shaping, and the like as each applies to the control of excessive eating. An early multiple case report by Stuart (1967; see also Stuart, 1971) established that the Ferster et al. procedure could yield rather large and stable weight losses—losses which were, in the words of one prominent reviewer, "the best ever reported for outpatient treatment of obesity . . ." (Stunkard, 1972, p. 393). Subsequent controlled investigations by Hagen (1974), Harris (1969), Harris and Bruner (1971), Penick et al. (1971), and Wollersheim (1970) consistently have demonstrated the superiority of the behavioral potpourri over a number of control and comparison procedures.

We are at once blessed with not one but *three* potentially effective treatment procedures for obesity. Do we separate and "choose our weapons," then, becoming therapeutic "respondent conditioners," "operant conditioners" or eclectic "potpourriers?" Whole schools of psychotherapeutic practice and thought have been founded on less data than there are on each of these treatment procedures. Or is it time for the development of general, guiding theories on which to base further research? These are questions which are dealt with by Hagen and Mahoney in their chapters in this book. We feel that the future of this important area is found within the conception of behavior therapy as an applied branch of experimental psychology.

BROADENING THE BASE OF BEHAVIOR THERAPY FOR OBESITY

The material in the preceeding section makes it clear that a variety of behavioral treatment procedures can be deployed with some success in the perennial battle of the bulge. We are still far, however, from being ready to develop complete intervention packages for widespread application. At the very least, much refinement is now in order. Prominent among current issues regarding the refinement of behavioral weight control procedures is the question: How can we broaden and thereby improve the empirical base of presently available treatments to include weight control procedures taken less directly from general behavior control manipulations (e.g., operant and respondent conditioning) and more directly from research bearing specifically on the processes of eating in the obese? The work of Stanley Schachter and his students and colleagues at Columbia University seems highly instrumental toward this end.

Stimulus Control and Weight Control

Seeking to further support and extend his observations on the role of cognitions in the experience of emotion, Schachter embarked on what was to be a long line of research on the eating processes of overweight and normal weight people (Schachter, 1967, 1968; Schachter, Goldman and Gordon, 1968). Several years of careful research have turned up a number of remarkably consistent facts about the eating processes of fat people (for documentary reviews, see Schachter, 1971a, 1971b). First, it was found that preloading or feeding solid foods to overweight students before an ad libitum eating situation had less of an effect on the amount of their eating than on normal students subjected to the same conditions. Related to this finding was the observation that injection of epinephrine, which inhibits gastric motility and increases blood sugar (both conditions being associated with low hunger levels), reduced the amount of food eaten by normal weight more than overweight subjects.

Of more direct interest to the behavior modifier, Schachter and his co-investigators have found that overweight volunteers tend to "eat by the clock" (i.e., when they perceive that it is their eating time), gauge their eating by food availability or the amount of food served, eat more of good and less of bad tasting food, eat less when aware of the amount of food eaten, and eat more and faster but less often (i.e., have fewer meals) than normals. Physiological processes associated with food deprivation and the sensation of hunger appear to be relatively unimportant. Instead, the eating behavior of overweight relative to normal weight people tends to be environmentally determined. Their eating is, in Schachter's words, stimulus bound; it tends to be triggered by external rather than internal (physiological) events.

These findings and others concerning the emotional reactivity, sensitivity to pain, and distractibility of overweight subjects have led Schachter and Rodin (1974) to view the obese as characteristically "external" in their interactions with the environment. They are, in a general predispositional sense, hyperresponsive to a variety of prominent stimuli or cues in their physical environment relative to normal and underweight people. In addition, the striking parallels between the behavior of overweight people and hyperphagic (super obese) rats with lesions in the ventromedial nuclei of their hypothalamus has led Schachter (see also Nisbett, 1968) to speculate that irregularities in this portion of the central nervous system are responsible for the excessive eating (and externality) of obese individuals. In particular, Schachter's feeling is that "functionally quiescent" ventromedial hypothalamic nuclei render obese people hyperresponsive to prominent stimuli in their environment, this hyperresponsivity leading to obesity in the case of food stimuli.

Theoretical speculations aside, there is much in Schachter's research of interest to the behavior therapist seeking to promote weight control in obese clients. Knowledge of the rudimentary processes whereby stimuli in the environment come to "control" certain aspects of behavior (see especially Terrace, 1966) makes it possible to consider stimulus control procedures as a potentially effective behavioral basis of weight loss treatment. Meaningful progress along this line has been made already by Mahoney (1972) and Stuart (1972). Further, a large group of investigators employing diverse treatment procedures have attempted to program "situational changes" in the eating and living environments of their overweight subjects. As yet, however, no one has attempted to develop and test a treatment for obesity which is emphatically oriented to stimulus control manipulations. This could be achieved easily by focusing on the characteristics of the overweight person's eating environment broadly conceptualized to include the grocery store, kitchen, and restaurant. Behavioral-environmental manipulations directed toward the reduction of food and eating cues would include shopping from a list, storing food out of sight, cooking with lids, serving buffet-style from the kitchen counter, quickly disposing of leftover food, and a score of similar, highly specific recommendations.

The Problem of Maintenance

The frequent and rapid return of newly lost excess poundage is a widely recognized phenomena. As Schachter and Rodin (1974) observe, "Almost any fat person can lose weight; few can keep it off" (p. 1).* Weight maintenance following treatment-induced weight losses appears to be no less a problem with behavioral treatments than it is with more traditional diet or exercise therapy.

Much of the problem in the maintenance of weight losses appears to center around the client's discontinuance of treatment-induced changes in eating and/or exercise. Upon completion of a course of treatment or reaching a desired weight level, clients often return to their old ways of doing things. Thus, they go off their reduction

---

* The bobbing up and down of body weight and associated waxing and waning of the weight loss effort has been called "the rhythm method of girth control" by noted nutritionist Jean Mayer.

diet, resume eating favored, high caloric foods, discontinue food records, cart the exercycle to the garage, and allow their health club membership to expire. Subsequently, lost pounds reappear. Were there no diet, exercise, reinforcement or conditioning regime to go off of, this might not be the case.

Weight loss within relatively permanent, stable dietary conditions can be achieved in two important ways. First, clients can be led to reduce caloric intake levels by eating less of everything within their own food choices as opposed to relying on a special or restricted diet for this purpose. Food preferences which develop rather early in life and reflect complex socio-economic influences are most difficult to change. Few people *like* being on a diet but most can live comfortably while eating less of what *they* do choose to eat. Second, treatment-instigated changes in food storage, preparation, and service habits that involve alteration of the eating environment (e.g., rearranging cupboards and refrigerator items; the use of new storage, preparation, and service dishes) in the interest of reducing food consumption will tend to persist beyond any formal treatment period. Behavior changes which are functionally linked to relatively stable changes in the environment will also prove to be relatively stable. Once again, then, the use of environmental or stimulus control procedures for weight control has a strong heuristic appeal.

Exporting Behavior Therapy for Obesity to Other Helping Professions

Few psychologists devote a substantial portion of their professional time to weight control problems other than their own. Nutritionists and dietitians do. Accordingly, it is probable that effective treatment procedures for obesity will gain widespread application through members of the latter professions, or, at the least, nutritionist-psychologist teams. This is good. The psychologist and nutritionist working together bring more to bear on problems of treatment and research than either alone (for a notable case in point see Stuart and Davis, 1972).

The opening move toward joint efforts should be made by the behavioral psychologist. Nutritionists should be invited to our research meetings, given extensive information on behavior therapy, and, generally, sought out as collaborators. They should then reciprocate. Training materials and procedures for the reciprocal education of nutritionists and psychologists should be developed and tested. The adequacy of the psychologists' nutritional counsel and efficacy of the nutritionists' behavioral treatment should be the object of careful study. The results of such a joint action relative to independent efforts should be reported in detail to members of both professions.

A STUDY OF TWO BEHAVIOR MODIFICATION PROCEDURES WITH NUTRITIONISTS AS THERAPISTS

Pursuant to the research questions detailed above, the current authors in conjunction with Drs. Ruth N. Lutz of the University of Missouri, Columbia, and May Bess Kohrs of Lincoln University undertook a comparison* of two behavioral weight loss procedures with nutritionists as therapists. The two treatments were: 1) a multiple principle, many technique based self-control treatment modeled after that used by Wollersheim (1970) and Hagen (1974), and much like that described by Harris (1969) and Penick et al. (1971); and 2) a self-control treatment package based almost exclusively on the principle and techniques of stimulus control. Treatment outcome measures taken immediately after treatment and 3, 6, 9, 12, and 18 months thereafter included total loss in body weight lost, percentage of unwanted weight lost, and percentage of excess weight lost.

Subjects

Fifty-four female volunteers from a small midwestern community served as subjects. This subject sample was taken from respondents to an advertisement in a local newspaper and radio announcements of a free weight reduction program being offered through hometown Lincoln University. Subjects were selected from the total group of volunteers, avoiding extremes in age and weight (selection age limits = 25 to 50; percentage overweight limits = 15 to 60 percent). No volunteers were accepted who had chronic health problems (e.g., diabetes) or had recently started

* This research was funded by USDA, Cooperative State Research Service Grant No. 316-15-16 awarded to Lincoln University, Jefferson City, Missouri.

or stopped taking medicine that could interfere with their reduction efforts (e.g., diuretics).

The final group of fifty-four subjects averaged 36.6 years of age ($SD = 8.1$), 178.4 pounds ($SD = 17.6$), and 39 percent overweight ($SD = 12.3$) as determined by the Metropolitan Life Insurance (1959) weight standards for women.

Therapists

The therapists were three female nutritionists, two with Ph.D.'s and the third with a M.S. degree in nutrition. Only the latter had any experience in behavior modification, having just completed her master's thesis in that area on the effectiveness of a self-control procedure in achieving weight losses in college age women (Kennedy, 1972). The nutritionist-therapists, competent to supply the nutrition information included in the treatment without special instruction, were trained in the behavior modification procedures with selected readings, detailed treatment manuals, and a number of instruction and question-and-answer briefing sessions. Each therapist conducted an equal number of groups in each treatment condition, one therapist conducting two and the other therapists one group in each of the two behavioral treatment conditions.

Treatment

Fifteen weekly treatment sessions lasting approximately one hour each were held in small groups of 5-8 subjects. The sessions were held in a large room containing a beam scale, bulletin board, blackboard, chairs, arranged in a semicircle, and an audio-visual taping machine, camera, and television monitor. All treatment sessions were videotaped for monitoring and training purposes, each session beginning with the subjects being weighed in front of the camera and examining themselves on the T.V. monitor. The expressed intent of both treatments was to teach subjects how to lose weight through reduced consumption of everything without the help of a special, restrictive diet. The specific nutrition and behavioral control lessons, subjects were told, would show them how this could be done.

"*Behavioral control*" (*Group BC*). This treatment was patterned after the weight-loss treatment described by Wollersheim (1970),

both being a conglomerate of several behavioral, self-control procedures. In addition, nutrition information was presented to subjects, with application to the control of eating. Included throughout
or at the various stages of this treatment were: a) a thorough consideration of the role and importance of a public and private commitment to weight loss; b) monitoring of daily food intake and
weekly weight changes with written records; c) social pressure
from the therapist and other group members on each subject to
continue and sustain weekly weight losses; d) instruction in specific, behavioral self-control techniques. Included among the latter
were principles of shaping, stimulus control, manipulation of deprivation and satiation, self-reward, response chaining, aversive
control and response substitution.

Presented alongside the self-control instruction were eleven nutrition lessons covering such topics as calories, food groupings, portion control, physical activity, food fads, proteins, vitamins and
minerals. As part of this nutritional aspect of treatment, subjects
were given calorie booklets and told to compute their daily caloric
intake from their daily food intake records. Thus, the goal of
treatment was to make subjects nutrition-wise as well as behaviorally self-controlling.

"Food management" (Group FM). This self-control weight loss
treatment drew almost exclusively from an external stimulus-con-
trol conceptualization of the overeater's problem suggested by the
work of Schachter and his associates. Self-control techniques within
this stimulus control focus were achieved in two important ways.
First, a "personal plate" and a "personal bowl," the use of which
was intended to increase the subjects' awareness of eating habits,
especially the frequency and amount of eating, were given to all
subjects. The six-ounce clear bowl and nine-inch dinner plate with
a wide rim were used throughout the fifteen weeks of treatment
within the following three rules: 1) everything that is eaten must
be eaten off the personal dishes; 2) the total amount of food to
be eaten at any one time must be put on the plate and/or bowl
before eating actually begins; 3) no seconds may be served to the
personal plate or bowl; once the initial serving of food is eaten,
eating is to stop.

In addition to the daily use of the personal dishes, subjects
received nine separate lessons on the "environmental control" of

eating at each of the various stages of the eating process. Thus, eating was discussed as it entails the buying, storing, cooking, serving and ingesting of food and the cleaning of the serving table and kitchen. Specific techniques to be used at each eating stage were presented each week in the form of a list of *Do's* and *Don'ts*, and included such suggestions as: a) *Do* buy groceries from a menu-based shopping list after a full meal; b) *Do* store all foods, especially refrigerator foods, in non-see-through containers; c) *Don't* hover over cooking food, being tempted to taste or eat it; d) *Don't* prepare or serve excessive amounts of food; e) *Don't* linger at the table or in the kitchen if you do not intend to eat; and f) *Do* eat reduced portions of all nutritious foods.

As in the Behavior Control treatment, subjects in this condition were frequently reminded of the importance of a commitment to weight loss, continuously monitored food intake and weight changes, and received weekly nutrition lessons. Calorie counting was optional with this group, and some subjects did, in fact, count or estimate daily caloric intake.

Delayed behavior control and food management treatment groups. Two groups of seven subjects, one to receive Behavior Control and the other Food Management treatment, were designated "Delayed Treatment" groups. These subjects, whose collective presence during the waiting period defines a no-treatment control group, went through the same pretreatment interviews and assessments as all other subjects, but began their treatment eight weeks after the other groups. Other than this delay, however, these subjects underwent the same Behavior Control and Food Management treatments as non-delayed subjects.

Procedure

At the time of their first telephone response to the public call for volunteers, it was determined whether a subject met the age and weight requirements. Sixty-six of 107 telephone inquiries so qualified and were given an initial interview. At that time a health and weight history was obtained, the program was explained, a participation-consent form was signed, and instructions were given to keep a three-day food record of everything eaten. Nine prospective subjects were eliminated for health reasons at the time of the initial interview and another three declined to participate. Within three weeks of the initial interview, all subjects were seen at the University of Missouri Low Level Radiation Laboratory, at which time they were weighed and body composition measures were taken. Within two weeks of this physical assessment, subjects were seen for a final pretreatment interview, their weights again being taken, the three-day food record collected, and scheduling for the 15 treatment sessions completed. Forty subjects randomly assigned to three Food Management and three Behavior Control therapy groups began treatment the following week. The remaining 14 subjects were assigned to the two Delayed Treatment groups and were told that, regrettably, the treatment groups were full and there would not be a nutritionist to work with them for eight weeks. All delayed-treatment subjects so informed were willing to wait through the delay and did so, receiving treatment thereafter.

At the time of the 15th and last treatment session, all subjects were given a Program Evaluation Questionnaire to fill out and return by mail. They were also provided a schedule of all the formal follow-up evaluations and encouraged to come in at these times to be weighed.

Results

A total of 43 subjects (including those in delayed treatment groups) completed the entire 14-week treatment program, leaving 23 subjects in Group BC and 20 in Group FM at the end of the treatment. The 11 treatment drop-outs, some of whom lost large amounts of weight, left the program for a variety of reasons, including personal and family health problems (4), pregnancy (1), marital problems (1), marriage during the program (1), and dissatisfaction with and/or poor success in the program (4). Of the 43 subjects completing the program, one had a hysterectomy and one a serious thyroid problem during the course of treatment (or delay) and were consequently lost to the study. Another subject who became pregnant immediately after completing her treatment was eliminated from the subsequent follow-up analyses.

Weight changes without treatment. As inspection of Figure 4-1 reveals, subjects' weights in all treatment conditons were highly stable during pretreatment and no-treatment delay periods. Thus, in the 2-4 week interval between the initial weigh-in and first

FIGURE 4-1
Mean Weight Losses for Delayed and Non-Delayed
Groups Before and After Treatment

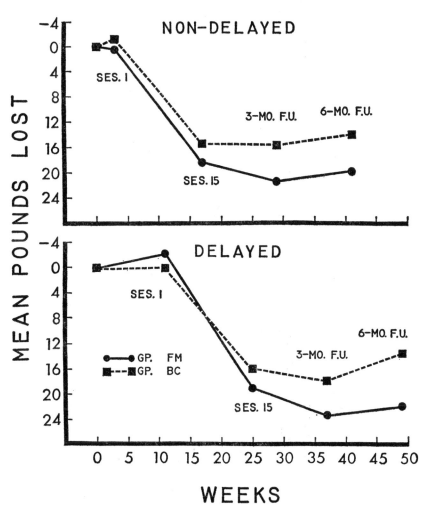

TABLE 4-1

Mean Weight Losses and Percentages of Success

Treatment		Total Pounds Lost			X% of Desired Loss*			X% of Excess Wt. Lost**		
		Post-Treatment	3 Mo. Follow-Up	6 Mo. Follow-Up	Post-Treatment	3 Mo. Follow-Up	6 Mo. Follow-Up	Post-Treatment	3 Mo. Follow-Up	6 Mo. Follow-Up
Food Management	X̄	18.6	22.0	20.4	64.4	52.1	47.8	41.1	47.8	43.9
	SD	7.6	9.7	10.1	32.3	25.5	25.4	21.3	23.2	22.9
	n	20	19	19	20	19	19	20	19	19
Behavior Control	X̄	16.1	17.0	14.6	60.1	52.3	45.4	36.9	38.5	32.0
	SD	4.9	7.0	8.8	27.7	31.3	35.1	17.7	22.1	23.5
	n	21	21	21	21	21	21	21	21	21
Total	X̄	17.4	19.4	17.4	62.2	52.2	46.6	38.9	42.9	37.7
	SD	6.4	8.6	9.8	29.7	28.3	30.5	19.4	22.8	23.7
	n	41	40	40	41	40	40	41	40	40

* $\sum_{1}^{n}$ Amount Lost/Amount Desired to Lose x 100 ÷ n

** $\sum_{1}^{n}$ Amount Lost/Amount Overweight x 100 ÷ n

TABLE 4-2

Number of Subjects in Three Weight Loss Categories
After 14 Weeks of Treatment

Treatment	0-13	14-28	>28
Food Management	6	11	3
Behavior Control	6	15	0

treatment session, subjects in non-delayed Groups BC and FM evidenced an average weight change of $+ 1.1$ ($SD = 4.3$) and $- .25$ ($SD = 3.7$) pounds, respectively. Similarly, subjects undergoing the 8-week treatment delay showed only minor weight fluctuations during a 10-12 week period (2-4 weeks pretreatment interval plus 8-week waiting period), with the mean change for delayed Groups BC and FM being 0.0 ($SD = 6.9$) and 2.2 ($SD = 2.9$) over the period of delay.

Weight losses following treatment. Statistical comparisons of both therapist and delay conditions within treatments reveal no therapist nor delay effects in either of the two therapeutic procedures. Accordingly, treatment groups were combined across therapists and delay conditions for all subsequent treatment group comparisons.

Large and highly significant weight losses were in evidence after 14 weeks of therapy in both behavioral treatment conditions (see Table 4-1), the distributions of weight losses in the treatment and no-treatment phases showing a very small amount of overlap. Subjects in Group FM lost an average of 18.6 lbs. ($SD = 7.6$) while those in Group BC lost an average of 16.1 lbs. ($SD = 4.9$), this difference being statistically non-significant. The two behavioral treatment procedures also evidenced comparable degrees of success on three additional weight loss indices: 1) mean percentage of desired reduction achieved, reflecting the amount of weight lost relative to weight loss goals set prior to treatment by each subject for post-treatment and follow-up time periods; 2) mean percentage of total *excess* weight lost as indicated by the Metropolitan Life Insurance (1959) weight standards for women; and, 3) number of subjects in three weight loss categories representing less than 1, 1-2, and 2 or more pounds lost per week during treatment (Table 4-2).

Weight losses at follow-up. At the time of the 3-month follow-up, subjects in Group FM had extended their weight losses
to an average of 22 lbs., sliding back only a pound and a half from
this to 20.4 total pounds off at the 6-month follow-up (see Table
4-1). Group BC did not fare quite so well at these two follow-ups,
but did post a respectable mean of 17.0 pounds lost at the 3-month
and 14.6 pounds lost at the 6-month follow-up. The differences
between the two behavioral treatment groups were significant at
both the 3-month (one-tailed t {38} = 1.85, $p < .05$) and 6-month
(one-tailed t {38} = 1.93, $p < .05$) follow-ups.

Statistical analysis of follow-up weights 9, 12, and 18 months
after treatment are not complete at this time, permitting only
partial reportage. Table 4-3 and Figure 4-2 reveal that weight
losses were maintained fairly well in both groups although the
stimulus control treatment posted better maintenance figures at all
points. Statistical comparisons of both groups at these points of follow-up contact failed to achieve significance despite what were at
times (see especially the 18-month point) large mean differences.
This is attributable to some extent to the large variance in weight
losses in Group BC ($SD - 16.21$). In this group one subject lost
40 and another *gained* 36 pounds during the follow-up period,
both scores being a standard deviation away from the next closest.
Although exclusion of these two subjects (whose weight changes
tend to cancel out each other) would greatly change the results
of the group comparison, such a procedure is not easily defended.

Attrition during the follow-up period tended to boost slightly
the mean weight losses for Group FM. Thus, the three "dropouts"
from Group BC included subjects both above and below the overall
mean weight loss for their group, but all the five subjects lost
from Group FM were below the mean for their group immediately
before leaving the study (i.e., they had lost less than others when
they dropped out).* The exact effect of this bias on group means
is beyond specification and most difficult to control for statistically.

Success predictors. Only two variables from a welter of self-
report data collected before treatment on weight history, eating
habits, activity level information, and family characteristics cor-

---

* Of the subjects who were lost during follow-up, three became pregnant,
three moved out of the state for vocational reasons, and two would not come in
for the final follow-up assessment.

TABLE 4-3

Mean Weight Losses for Each Therapy Condition
9, 12, and 18 Months After Treatment

	TREATMENT					
Months of Follow-Up		BC			FM	
	x̄	SD	N	x̄	SD	N
9	12.85	11.48	20	16.66	9.64	18
12	12.75	13.99	20	13.76	9.79	17
18	8.27	16.21	18	15.33	10.42	15

FIGURE 4-2

Mean Weight Losses for Each Therapy Group at End of
Treatment (EOT) and During Follow-up

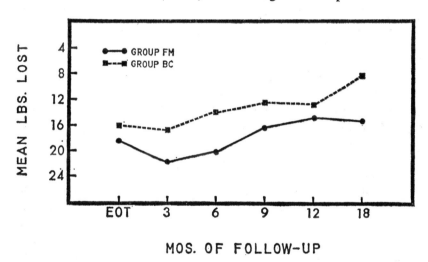

related significantly with subjects' weight losses at the end of treatment. The two potential success predictors are the related ones of proportion of life overweight (number of years overweight relative to age) and age of onset of overweight; they correlate $(r) — .47$ $(p < .01)$ and $.44$ $(p < .01)$ respectively with the absolute amount of weight loss immediately after treatment.

Discussion of Findings

These results show that a behavioral treatment procedure emphasizing the elimination or reduction of eating cues in the obese person's environment can have significant and lasting treatment effects. The superiority of the stimulus control treatment over a more combination-of-ingredients approach during follow-up may result from the: a) direct and *focal* relevance of stimulus control manipulations to the control of eating; b) clarity and ease with which the stimulus control procedures were programmed into specific behavioral guidelines, often of a detailed "do" or "don't do" nature; and c) relative permanence of environmental-behavioral changes (e.g., rearranging cupboards, storing foods in non-see-through containers, eating less of preferred foods) made within the stimulus control rationale and the resultant alignment of the conditions of maintenance with the conditions of behavior change (i.e., weight loss). The last of these possibilities as an explanation of the superior maintenance of weight losses in the stimulus control treatment has relevance to the general issue of the stability and generalizability of treatment-induced behavior changes. The first offers support to Schachter's observation that overweight people tend to be externally "bound" in regard to their eating behavior.

The weight reductions achieved herein with nutritionists are equal or superior to those produced by a number of behavioral psychologists using treatment procedures both similar to and different from those we used. The failure of an earlier, unaided effort to produce meaningful weight losses with a behavioral treatment by one of the current investigators (Kennedy, 1972) in contrast to the present results suggests that training, guidance and ongoing consultation in the principles and procedures of behavior therapy are necessary if sizable and stable weight reductions are to achieved. It has already been emphasized that the skills and knowledge of nutritionists are indispensable to nutritionally and medically sound weight control. The present study attests, then, to both the importance and feasibility of joint psychologist-nutritionist efforts in treatment and research on weight control.

SUGGESTIONS FOR FUTURE RESEARCH

This line of research is currently being extended in two additional research projects. First, the same basic stimulus control treatment package has been used by 8 extension home economists working in four areas in the state of Missouri to treat 110 clinically obese women. At the end of 20 weeks of treatment (subjects are currently in the follow-up phase), the mean weight loss for all participants was 17.6 pounds. This figure is comparable to that obtained at the end of treatment in the first study and constitutes replication of that research finding in a wholly applied setting. Second, a project is currently under way extending these techniques to obese *families* seeking help in weight loss and control as a family unit. This latter experimental effort has implications for early direction, treatment, and prevention of obesity that are of fundamental importance.

The following additional issues and trends in research on the behavioral management of obesity are suggested by the foregoing material:

1) Few weight loss programs, behavioral or otherwise, have produced "graduates" capable of continuing to lose weight after formal treatment is over. Once treatment ends, body weight either stabilizes or increases. What is needed to counteract this is either extended treatment which ends when subjects attain their ideal weight or programming helpful in extending weight losses *after* a period of regular and frequent treatment sessions. Along the latter lines, we are now comparing post-treatment booster contacts of a fading (i.e., decreasingly frequent) or regular interval (i.e., monthly) nature over a 12-month period with 94 of the treated obese women referred to earlier.

2) The current emphasis on weight *loss* should give way to a more complete focus on weight *control*. Weight losses which are not maintained over extended periods of time are of little nutritional or medical value. Further, they may undermine future weight loss efforts. Treatment which produces sizable weight losses which are not maintained is no longer noteworthy. Twelve-month follow-up data on experimentally treated subjects should be reported as routine.

It is likely that progress toward weight control as a lifetime habit will depend on broad treatment and follow-up programs emphasizing nutrition, behavioral programming and regular exercise. The last of these elements has been ignored for the most part by behavior therapists, though considered important by most nutritionists (especially Mayer, 1968).

3) All fat people are not alike in their corpulence. Mayer (1968), for instance, has identified five causal types of obesity in man—genetic, hypothalmic, non-hypothalmic central nervous systemic, endocrinologic, and other (e.g., socio-cultural). These etiological factors as well as the potentially important distinction between juvenile and adult onset obesity (Grinker, 1973) have been ignored by most treatment investigators. In a behavioral sphere, it may be possible to classify fat people by eating type such as volume, problem food, and non-distributive eaters, and tailor treatment more carefully to their particular type of eating disturbance. Where eating habits are not at fault, increased exercise should become the focus of treatment. Research along these lines is currently under way at the University of Missouri.

4) The focus of many behavioral weight control procedures has been on the conditions surounding the initiation ("start mechanism") of eating. This is consistent with Schachter's observation that fat people (like hyperphagic rats) eat in response to eating cues in their environment, notably the sight, taste, and availability of food. Overlooked to a large extent has been the observation (e.g., Schachter and Rodin, 1974) that obese humans and rats eat no more often than their normal weight counterparts, but eat *more* when they do eat. This suggests that at least some obese organisms suffer a defect in the "stop mechanism" of eating. Once they start eating, for whatever reasons, they tend to eat beyond the point that normal weight organisms stop. This speculation and its implications for the function and role of the lateral and ventromedial nuclei of the hypothalamus in eating (and the occurrence of emotional responses) merit independent and detailed attention which cannot be given here. Whether empirically supported at this time or not, however, the focus on the *termination* of ongoing eating processes is relatively new in the treatment of obesity and opens up important new potentials for the behavioral intervention of this problem within the "applied research" conception of behavior therapy described earlier.

Chapter 5

Effect of Deposit Contracts and Distractibility on Weight Loss and Maintenance

John P. Vincent, Lois Schiavo,
and Ronald Nathan

In recent years, self-management approaches to the treatment of obesity have become increasingly popular. Since the first reports of their use by Ferster, Nurnberger, and Levitt (1962), an impressive armamentarium of self-management techniques have been developed to teach appropriate eating habits, establish situational control over eating behavior, and strike a proper balance between energy intake and energy expenditure. The development of training procedures for weight management has been accompanied by numerous research studies demonstrating their efficacy. Despite the methodological shortcomings inherent in many of these studies, self-management approaches for obesity have generally been found to: 1) be effective for most clients in achieving weight loss during treatment (Harris, 1969; Penick et al., 1971; Stuart, 1967, 1971; Wollersheim, 1970), 2) owe their effectiveness to factors other than non-specific treatment effects (Wollersheim, 1970; Stuart, 1971; Abrahms and Allen, 1974), and 3) be somewhat more effective than other treatment modalities (Wollersheim, 1970; Jeffrey, 1972; Penick et al., 1971).

There are at least two issues which appear unresolved. First, high variability in weight loss is associated with most self-management programs. For some subjects, dramatic weight losses are obtained during treatment, whereas for other subjects, minimal weight losses are achieved (Penick et al., 1971; Harris and Bruner, 1971). In the present study, findings from the social psychological laboratory concerning the stimulus binding hypothesis (Rodin, 1973) provided a potential predictor variable to weight loss in self-management programs emphasizing restructuring of situational stimulus control over eating behavior. Second, as with most treatments for obesity, many subjects in self-management programs fail to maintain their weight loss (Hagen, 1974; Harris and Bruner, 1971; Hall, 1972; Mahoney, 1974). External inducements, in particular deposit contracts, have been an integral part of many of the self-management programs. However, their potentially adverse effects on maintenance of weight loss have not been satisfactorily investigated.

Differential Effectiveness

Variability in response to self-management procedures has been a problem reported by many investigators. Penick et al. (1971) noted that ". . . both the best and worst results were obtained in these [behavior modification] groups" (p. 54). The consistent finding of differential effectiveness in response to self-management of obesity (Horan and Johnson, 1971; Mahoney, 1974; Harris and Bruner, 1971) raises the need for useful predictor variables to identify those subjects who will succeed and those subjects who will fail. A promising variable in this regard is the stimulus boundedness of obese subjects. Beginning in the late fifties, numerous investigators have noted that obese subjects tend to be less responsive to internal sensations of hunger and satiation, and more responsive to a variety of external stimuli than non-obese subjects. Relative to non-obese subjects, obese subjects have been shown to report hunger independent of gastric contractions (Stunkard, 1959), eat more when presented with experimentally induced time sets of "dinner time" (Schachter and Gross,1968), report hunger independent of time since last meal (Nisbett, 1968), eat more when food is visible (Ross, 1970; Nisbett, 1968), and are generally more influenced by the taste of food (Hashim and Van Tallie, 1965). The findings concerning the external stimulus boundedness of obese subjects has been extended beyond food related cues in several studies (Rodin, Herman, and Schachter, 1972; Rodin, 1973). In Rodin's (1973) extension, the proofreading accuracy of obese and non-obese subjects under conditions of distraction (competing auditory cues) and no distraction (silence) was investigated. Compared with non-obese subjects, the performance of obese subjects was superior in the no distraction condition and inferior in the distraction condition.

The consistent findings concerning external stimulus boundedness have direct implications for self-management programs which emphasize restructuring the situational control of eating. Tactics such as using smaller dinnerware, removing forbidden foods from the household, and restricting eating to one location (McReynolds et al., 1974; Stuart and Davis, 1972) are all consonant with the notion that obese individuals must modify external food-related stimuli which impinge upon their senses in order to achieve weight loss.

It may be further reasoned that responsiveness to external stimuli is not only a dimension which discriminates obese from non-obese subjects, but is also an individual difference variable which is normally distributed within the obese population. The extent to which an obese subject is responsive to external cues may be an important predictive factor which is related to success in a self-management obesity program.

Maintenance

The maintenance of weight loss is the ultimate goal of any treatment for obesity. Although many self-management programs have reported favorable maintenance effects at follow-up (Penick et al., 1971; Wollersheim, 1970; Stuart, 1971), the failure of many subjects to sustain weight loss is a recurrent finding (Hall, 1972; Harris and Bruner, 1971; Mahoney, 1974). Numerous factors may be isolated which favorably affect weight maintenance, such as motivation of subjects (Jeffrey, 1974), change in eating habits (Mahoney, 1974), and programming support from significant others in the subject's social environment (Abrahms and Allen, 1974). However, questions can be raised concerning which elements of self-management programs adversely affect weight maintenance.

The use of external inducements (deposit contracts) may be postulated as one treatment component which mitigates against successful weight maintenance. Despite the widespread use of deposit contracts in self-management programs (Harris and Bruner, 1971; Jeffrey, 1974; Mann, 1972; Mahoney, Moura, and Wade, 1973; Abrahms and Allen, 1974), questions can be raised of both a procedural and theoretical nature.

At a procedural level, there is some disagreement as to whether the deposit should be used as a self-reward, by returning the subject's money in small increments to reinforce progress, or as a self-punishment, by penalizing subjects in similar amounts for violations of the program. Findings by Mahoney et al. (1973) suggest that the self-reinforcement model or self-reinforcement plus self-punishment may be more effective than self-punishment alone; however, the issue is by no means resolved. In fact, the distinction may be an artificial one in that penalizing oneself for violations of the program or electing not to reward oneself may have the same net effect. Few guidelines exist with respect to the behaviors upon which a deposit is made contingent. Monetary contingencies may be placed upon attending sessions and completing weigh-ins (Abrahms and Allen, 1974), upon dropping out of the program (Jeffrey, 1974), upon restructuring eating habits (Mahoney, 1974), upon actual weight loss (Mann, 1972), or upon both habit change and weight loss (Mahoney et al., 1973). Some evidence was reported by Mann (1972) that placing contingencies upon actual weight loss may encourage subjects to adopt extreme measures such as taking laxatives or diuretics, and engaging in vigorous exercise before weighing in order to lose weight rapidly and avoid the aversive consequences of forfeiting money. A final procedural question involves how much money the client deposits, and whether this amount is a flat fee or adjusted to the subject's financial resources. Differences in the amount of deposit range from $10.00 to $35.00, and in one study (Mann, 1972) clients were encouraged to deposit a valuable or prized possession. When a flat fee is used, as opposed to a percentage of clients' income, one encounters a problem in the differential impact of the deposit across groups. A flat fee may unfairly penalize subjects from a low socioeconomic level, yet may have limited impact on a person from a higher economic level. Taken collectively, the procedural discrepancies in the literature make comparisons among studies and interpretation of findings extremely difficult.

At a theoretical level, one may also wonder what effect deposits have on weight maintenance once the money has been returned. Without some continuing form of external inducement it is reasonable to expect that clients will return to their former pattern of eating too much, exercising too little, and gaining weight. This concern is bolstered by laboratory findings from attribution theorists who have shown that behavior changes attributed to oneself are maintained better than behavior changes attributed to an external agent (Storms and Nisbett, 1970; Davison and Valins, 1969; Davison, Tsujimoto and Glaros, 1973). With deposit contracts, do clients attribute their weight loss to an external agent (monetary inducement) and will such an attribution have an adverse effect on weight maintenance in the clinical context? Previous research on the use of deposit contracts for weight management (Jeffrey, 1974; Abrahms and Allen, 1974) does not answer this question since, in both studies cited, the monetary inducement was provided at follow-up. Thus, the possibility remains that once the deposit is completely returned, weight loss will no longer be maintained and long-term behavior change may be sacrificed in favor of short-term gains.

Overview of Present Studies

In order to investigate the predictive relationship of stimulus boundedness to successful weight loss and the impact of deposit contracts on weight loss and maintenance, two studies were conducted. The first study was a partial replication of Rodin's (1973) study comparing obese and non-obese females in terms of proof-reading accuracy under conditions of distraction and no distraction. The present study was an attempt to extend Rodin's findings beyond college males to a sample of females recruited from the community. Within the obese sample, the predictive utility of distractibility was also assessed in terms of its possible relationship to successful weight loss. The Rodin study was seen as particularly well suited to the present need since it circumvented the methodological problems associated with the use of food-related external cues.

Study two dealt with the impact of deposit contract versus no-deposit contract on both weight loss and weight maintenance. Furthermore, the assignment of obese subjects to one or two therapists, under either deposit or no-deposit conditions, allowed investigation of therapist skill and personal attributes in relation to treatment efficacy.

METHOD

Design

Figure 5-1 presents the experimental design for the two-phase study. Phase one represents a partial replication of Rodin's (1973) study in which the proofreading accuracy of obese and non-obese subjects was compared under conditions of distraction and no distraction from competing auditory stimuli. Phase two represents a self-management treatment study in which the obese subjects were randomly assigned to one of two therapists, under one of two conditions: deposit or no-deposit. The main dependent variables were pounds lost, reduction index of weight loss, and body density compared at pre, post, and 2-month follow-up. Various predictors of success in the weight reduction program were also examined.

Subjects

Thirty-four obese female subjects were recruited from the Houston community through physician referral and posters announcing the opening of a therapy-research program for the treatment of obesity. To be eligible for the project, subjects were required to be: 1) at least 20 percent overweight based upon Metropolitan Life Insurance norms for females (1973), 2) between 18 and 40 years of age, 3) living with someone who would be willing to serve as a co-participant for purposes of obtaining reliability checks on self-reported data, 4) willing to participate in "one brief study" which was described as unrelated to the treatment program and which supposedly dealt with the "physiological and psychological effects of sensory overload," 5) willing to participate in follow-up sessions at two months, six months, and one year, 6) willing to pay $5.00 for necessary materials and a deposit of 5 percent of net monthly combined income (which

FIGURE 5-1
General Experimental Design for Study 1 and Study 2

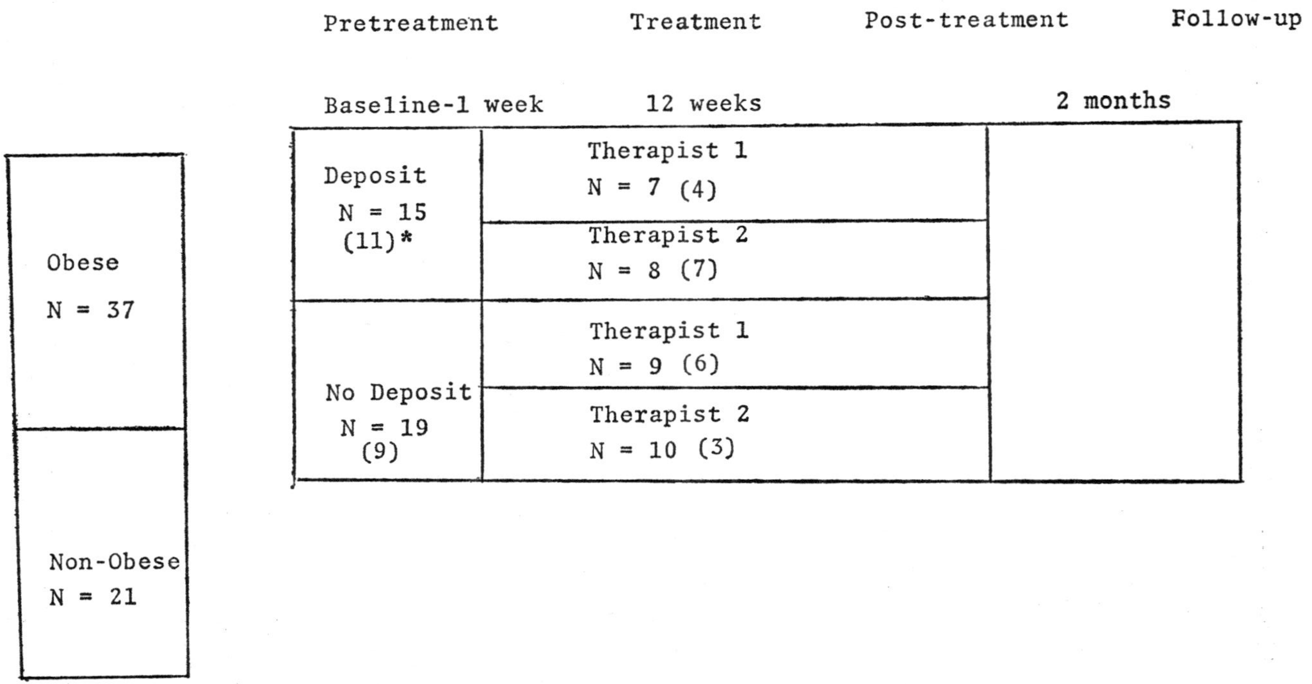

Pretreatment	Treatment	Post-treatment	Follow-up
Baseline-1 week	12 weeks	2 months	

Deposit
N = 15
(11)*

Therapist 1
N = 7 (4)

Therapist 2
N = 8 (7)

No Deposit
N = 19
(9)

Therapist 1
N = 9 (6)

Therapist 2
N = 10 (3)

Obese
N = 37

Non-Obese
N = 21

* Number that completed program.

would be completely refundable upon following specified steps of the program), 7) not involved in any other treatment for obesity, and 8) willing to obtain a physician's statement that the subject was physically able to participate in the program. The obese sample was an average of 31 years of age (S.D. = 7 years), 51 percent overweight (S.D. = 22 percent), had 14 years of education (S.D. = 2 years), came from a socio-economic level of 2.7 (S.D. = 1.8) based upon the Hollingshead-Redlich nine-point index (Hollingshead and Redlich, 1958). In terms of marital status, 65 percent were married, 15 percent were single, 20 percent were divorced. Full-time employment was reported by 60 percent of the sample. Previous professional help for obesity had been sought by 75 percent of the sample, 55 percent had joined weight reducing clubs, 45 percent had sought both professional help and joined clubs, and 15 percent sought no outside assistance for their weight problem.

Twenty-one non-obese volunteer female subjects were also recruited by newspaper advertisements and word-of-mouth to conduct the replication of Rodin's (1973) study. To be eligible for participation in the study, non-obese subjects were required to be: 1) within 10 percent of desirable weight as defined by the Metropolitan Life Insurance norms for females (1973), 2) between 18 and 40 years of age, 3) not living alone, and 4) willing to participate in "one brief study on the physiological and psychological effects of sensory overload."

The non-obese sample was recruited from community sectors at the same socioeconomic level as the obese sample, although no attempt was made to match groups on specific demographic variables.

Dependent Measures

Height and weight. Height and weight were measured to the nearest inch and nearest pound, respectively, in street clothing and without shoes on a standard physician's balance scale. Indices of weight loss included pounds lost, percentage of body weight lost, and a reduction index which controlled for differences in initial weight, target weight, and weight loss. The reduction index suggested by Feinstein (1959) is obtained by the following formula:

$$\text{Reduction Index} = \text{Weight lost} \; \frac{\text{Initial Weight}}{\text{Surplus Weight} \times \text{Target}} \; \times \; 100$$

Target weight was defined as the ideal weight for the subject's height according to the Metropolitan Life Insurance norms.

Body density. To provide a measure of body density, which is highly related to lean body mass, caliper measurements were obtained at 3 body sites, and combined according to the procedures outlined by Pollock et al. (in press) to arrive at a single index. Previous research has indicated that this body density index is highly correlated with body density measures obtained in underwater weighings. An increase in body density would be expected in a successful weight reduction program.

Distractibility. An index of stimulus boundedness was obtained according to procedures outlined by Rodin (1973), but modified to control for the subject's ability to proofread. The distractibility score was calculated by subtracting the percentage of errors in the distraction condition from the percentage of errors in the no-distraction condition on the Rodin (1973) proofreading task.

Additional Measures

Predictor variables. As part of the pre-treatment assessment battery, three additional measures were included as potential predictors to success in the treatment program: the Rotter locus of control scale (Rotter, 1966), the Eysenck neuroticism scale (Eysenck, 1964), and the Marlowe-Crowne scale of social desirability (Crowne and Marlowe, 1964). The distractibility score obtained in the partial replication of Rodin's (1973) study was also treated as a predictor variable in the analyses of weight loss in the obese sample.

Self-monitoring data. A series of self-monitoring forms were adapted from Stuart and Davis (1972) or were specially designed for the present study. Although these forms were not specifically used as dependent measures, these forms assessed the subject's compliance with various aspects of the treatment program. They included a baseline eating habits form; graphs of weight, caloric intake, and exercise (measured in caloric units of expenditure); and a self-management curriculum checklist which accompanied each step of the treatment program. Subjects completed the checklist on the morning, afternoon, and evening of each day and placed a check by those elements of the program which they had followed, those which they had not followed, and those which did not apply that day. Reliability estimates of this self-recorded data were obtained twice per week from the designated co-participant who noted on a signed form the subject's morning weight and whether or not the specified program had been followed.

Therapists. Two male graduate students served as therapists. Therapist 1 was a second year graduate student in clinical psychology whose theoretical orientation was in line with a social learning framework. Therapist 2 was a graduate student in philosophy who had completed 15 hours of advanced clinical psychology training seminars, and whose orientation was eclectic. Both therapists had a minimum of 12 months supervised group psychotherapy experience and underwent 14 hours of intensive training in the treatment of obesity beginning 4 weeks prior to the first treatment session. Detailed outlines of each treatment session were provided and roleplaying and feedback, as well as direct instruction, were used in the training phase. All treatment sessions were videotape recorded and discussed at weekly supervision meetings conducted by a Ph.D. clinical psychologist.

To control for confounding of the therapist's skill, personal attributes, and theoretical orientation, with the major experimental manipulation, each therapist treated one group in the deposit condition and one group in the no-deposit condition. The therapists were also kept blind as to the nature of the investigation and hypotheses of the study.

Treatment Groups

Subjects were randomly assigned from stratified blocks (percentage overweight) to one of four experimental groups: 1) therapist 1, no-deposit; 2) therapist 1, deposit; 3) therapist 2, no-deposit; 4) therapist 2, deposit. Each group was treated using a standard self-management program adapted from Stuart and Davis (1972) for ten sessions over a thirteen-week period of time. A description of the curriculum for each session will be presented below.

Deposit condition. Subjects were required to post a deposit of 5 percent of the net monthly income per family. This deposit was contingent upon attendance, punctuality, completion of weekly data forms, and specific habit change exercises prescribed each session. The habit change exercises included restructuring the stimuli associated with eating behavior, caloric intake restriction, and a gradual program to increase energy expenditure. Consecutive violations of the prescribed rules resulted in forfeiture of 1/10, 2/10, 3/10, and 4/10 of the deposit, which was forwarded to a non-profit charity organization. The fifth violation of the program would have resulted in termination of treatment; however, the maximum number of violations was three. The terms of the deposit were presented in a written contract which was signed by subject and therapist, and specified the return of all unused funds following the last treatment session. Subjects in the deposit condition were also presented with a rationale stressing the necessity of an external inducement to encourage compliance with the program. The external attribution rationale was reiterated when appropriate during the course of treatment.

No-deposit condition. Subjects were given the same treatment rules as those in the deposit condition and required to sign a written contract to acknowledge acceptance of those rules. However, no monetary deposit was required, and there was no contingency placed upon violations of the program. Since all subjects had been told during the phone contact that a deposit would be required (to insure comparability of groups at baseline), they were given a rationale stressing the importance of internal factors such as self-determination, hard work, and earnest effort. The internal attribution rationale was reiterated when necessary.

Stimulus Materials for Distractibility Task

The replication of Rodin's (1973) study incorporated proofreading texts and distraction audio tapes closely resembling the stimulus materials used in the original study. The four proofreading passages were taken from Jacob's *The Death and Life of Great American Cities* (1961), and written so that each passage contained approximately the same number and variety of errors. Two 10-minute audio distraction tapes were made from verbatim transcripts of the original tapes. Tape one asked the subject to relax and think about rain. A soothing female voice then poetically described the properties of rain as they would be perceived by the five senses, and traced some of the symbolic associations one might make while experiencing rain. For example, the subject was asked to "think of how you run, sometimes, to get out of rain, and no matter how fast you run, you can never keep time with the rapid cadence of the thousands of millions of raindrops. The rain comes on you like a great cleansing thing. . . ."

Tape two asked the subject to relax and think about seashells. It described in a way similar to tape one the properties and associations of seashells. For example, the subjects was asked to "remember how, when you were a child, you went hunting for seashells along the beach and how you gathered so many different kinds and sizes? Remember how exciting it was to shake the sand off a shell and find that you had picked up a perfect shell. . . ."

PROCEDURE

Initial contact. Subjects responding to posters or referred by private physicians were initially contacted for a phone interview. The program was briefly described as a ten-session therapy-research program emphasizing restructuring of eating habits, sound nutrition, and increasing energy expenditure. At this time, subjects were told that the program would not make use of fad diets, drugs, or any quick-weight-loss schemes, but rather an individualized program designed to be used over an extended period of time. After subjects expressed a desire to participate, dates and times were scheduled for the study 2 to 3 weeks prior to the beginning of the treatment sessions. Referrals were offered to those subjects who did not meet the screening criteria.

Study 1

The first study was a partial replication of Rodin's study (1973). The subject read an introduction to the experiment which began, "Thank you for coming in today. This is an experiment having to do with stimulation of several sense organs simultaneously. . . ." The experimenter explained that the physiological measurement is meaningless without knowledge of a person's height and weight, and that the primary data source was the galvanic skin response. The subject was informed that a measurement of her baseline galvanic skin response would be taken and electrodes were attached to the subject's wrists. At this point the subject was instructed to add columns of numbers while an ohm meter apparently "measured" her galvanic skin response.

The subject was then told, "Your primary task is to attend to the visual monitoring, but at the same time you will be listening to auditory material so that we may uniformly control each subject's stimulus input." Furthermore, the subject was told to proofread by underlining each error and "placing a check in the margin next to the line where the error appears." The subject randomly received one of the four passages from Jacob's *The Death and Life of Great American Cities* (1961). A tape recorder was started and the subject had ten minutes of silence before hearing instructions to remove her headphones and to underline the last sentence proofed. Following this, a second "baseline" was taken. The subject then proofread another randomly chosen selection while hearing one of the two distraction tapes.

After the second proofreading task, the subjects were debriefed by the experimenter in the following way. The subjects were asked if they had any questions. If so, the questions were answered by the most appropriate of the following ploys: (a) "I am only a research assistant and don't really know, but it is an interesting question," (b) "That's a very interesting hypothesis, what made you think of that?" or (c) "We are only interested in group scores, so I don't think I could ever tell you your own results. Even the group results will not be available until the data have been analyzed." The non-obese were offered the opportunity to receive a copy of the results after the study was over. The obese subjects were then told that the Obesity Clinic left a message with the experimenter to the effect that the clinic would be calling them in the next three weeks to start treatment. All subjects were asked not to discuss the experiment with anyone at any time and were thanked for their participation.

The ten treatment sessions were conducted over a thirteen-week period, and were adopted from Stuart and Davis' treatment program as outlined in *Slim Chance in a Fat World* (1972). In general, each session placed emphasis on situational control, i.e., identifying and modifying environmental cues associated with problematic eating, and a balance between caloric intake and energy expenditure.

Session I. Session I was primarily concerned with introductory information on obesity and stressed the importance of baseline recording. Instruction in the use of self-monitoring forms, an exercise plan, and graphs were given to all clients. A research assistant obtained the client's pre-treatment height, weight, and body density measures. The subject's weight was obtained for each session thereafter.

Session II. Expectations for the clients about treatment were explained, and subjects were given their respective deposit, no-deposit instructions. The terms of treatment were specified in a deposit contract (treatment contract for no-deposit subjects) and signed by all subjects. The initial rules in situational control were presented in an attempt to help clients gain control over the antecedents associated with problematic eating. Individual caloric requirements were calculated and the rudiments of an exercise program were introduced. The food exchange program was presented along with an introduction to the principles of nutrition upon which the exchange program was based.

In the week following Session II, the designated co-participants were contacted and instructed to complete signed reliability forms on the self-monitored data.

Session III. Additional strategies of situational control were presented which included how to shop for food and ways to avoid problematic food. The necessity of avoiding undue sleep, activity, and food deprivation was stressed, and myths about dieting were discussed. A formal exercise program was initiated in which caloric expenditure was gradually increased by roughly twenty-five calories each day. This program was continued throughout treatment until a realistic exercise goal was achieved.

Session IV. Additional situational control rules were prescribed to increase the response cost associated with eating by lengthening the chain of behaviors, make eating less "automatic," and offer the client several choice points whether or not to eat. The concepts of reprogramming the social environment and social reinforcement were also introduced. Techniques to modify eating responses were offered which, in turn, would foster a "feeling of self-control." The problems involved in extending situational control to parties and restaurants were discussed, and subjects were instructed to plan a practice trip to a restaurant.

Session V. Potential problems and solutions for the impending Christmas holidays were explored, and the information on nutrition and situational control was reiterated.

Session VI. Three weeks had transpired between Session V and Session VI.

Clients were encouraged to share their experiences and insights gleaned over the holiday period. Furthermore, to clarify the relationship between setting, eating, and reinforcement, clients pinpointed the antecedents, responses, and consequences of their own eating behavior. The importance of sound nutrition and consistent exercises were underscored.

Sessions VII to X. Individual requirements for long-term weight management were realistically appraised with respect to: 1) situational control of eating, 2) caloric intake, 3) energy expenditure, and 4) development of non-food recreational outlets. At Session X, post treatment body density measures were obtained.

Follow-up

After two months, all subjects were scheduled to obtain measures of weight, body density, and their perceptions of the treatment program.

RESULTS

Data collected during the distractibility study (Study One) and during pre, post, and follow-up time periods of the treatment study (Study Two) were analyzed with respect to the major a priori experimental hypotheses. Results from the distractibility study were analyzed with t tests of mean group differences between obese and non-obese subjects. The effects of general self-management treatment procedures and specific deposit and no-deposit manipulations on weight loss and weight maintenance were assessed with multiple t tests, non-parametric tests, and two-way analyses of variance using the main dependent variables of pounds lost, reduction index, and body density. Supplemental correlational analyses were then performed to determine any relationship be-

TABLE 5-1
Rodin's (1973) "Mean Proofreading Accuracy: Number Correct/Number Possible on Pages Read"

Subjects	No Distraction	Neutral Distraction	Difference (No Distraction-Distraction)
Obese	.612	.469	+.143
Non-obese	.471	.514	—.043

For no distraction, obese vs. non-obese t = 2.62, p < .02. For obese no distraction vs. neutral distraction t = 2.66, p < .02. Variance based on mean square error term for the "distraction" analysis of variance and both p values reported are two-tailed.

tween various predictor variables and success in the treatment program as defined by the reduction index scores.

Distractibility (Study One)

Proofreading accuracy scores were obtained for obese and non-obese subjects by subtracting the percentage of errors identified in the distraction condition from the errors found in the no-distraction condition. Table 5-1 presents the mean proofreading accuracy scores from Rodin's (1973) original study. As can be seen, obese subjects identified 61 percent of the errors under no-distraction, 47 percent errors under distraction, for a difference of X = +14 percent between conditions. Non-obese subjects identified 47 percent errors under no-distraction, 51 percent under distraction, for a difference of —4 percent between conditions. A t test on group means from the Rodin study had revealed significant differences between groups under the no-distraction condition, and an analysis of variance had revealed a significant subject × condition interaction. Table 5-2 presents the mean proofreading accuracy scores obtained in the present study. A slight (non-significant) decrement in proofreading accuracy was found for obese subjects between the no-distraction and distraction conditions (means = 60 percent, 59 percent, respectively, for a difference of +1 percent). Contrary to the original study, non-obese subjects also evidenced a slight (non-significant) decrement in proofreading accuracy between no-distraction and distraction conditions (means = 63 percent, 58 percent, respectively, for a

TABLE 5-2

Study I: "Mean Proofreading Accuracy: Number
Correct/Number Possible on Pages Read"

Subjects	No Distraction	Neutral Distraction	Difference (No distraction-distraction)
Obese	.605	.592	+.013
Non-obese	.629	.581	—.048

For no distraction, obese vs. non-obese t = .759 (opposite direction) nonsignificant. For obese, no distraction vs. neutral distraction t = .553 (expected direction nonsignificant. The first "t" is a t test for unequal standard deviations, the second is a t test for matched data.

difference of 5 percent). Statistical analyses of these data using t tests revealed no significant differences between or within groups across conditions (see Figure 5-2). A part correlation between obese and non-obese subjects on proofreading accuracy under the distraction condition (with proofreading accuracy in the no-distraction condition held constant) revealed a non-significant correlation of .10 in the direction opposite to that predicted. These findings represent a failure to replicate the original findings by Rodin (1973). Additional correlational analyses were performed to investigate whether the subject's educational level was significantly related to performance under the two conditions and thereby constituted a confounding variable. For the obese subjects, non-significant correlations between educational level and performance under distraction ($r = .25$) and between educational level and performance under no-distraction ($r = .15$) ruled out this possibility.

Effects of Treatment Procedures (Study Two)

Random assignment. Attrition of 14 subjects yielded 7 subjects in therapist 1-deposit group, 4 in therapist 2-deposit group, 3 in therapist 1-no-deposit, and 6 in therapist 2-no-deposit. T tests on demographic variables and dependent measures indicated that compared with subjects who remained in treatment, dropouts were not significantly different on any of 11 variables, except level of education. Dropouts had significantly fewer years of education than those who remained in treatment (mean = 13, 14.5, respec-

FIGURE 5-2

Graph of Proofreading Accuracy Data from Rodin's (1973) Study and the Partial Replication (Study I)

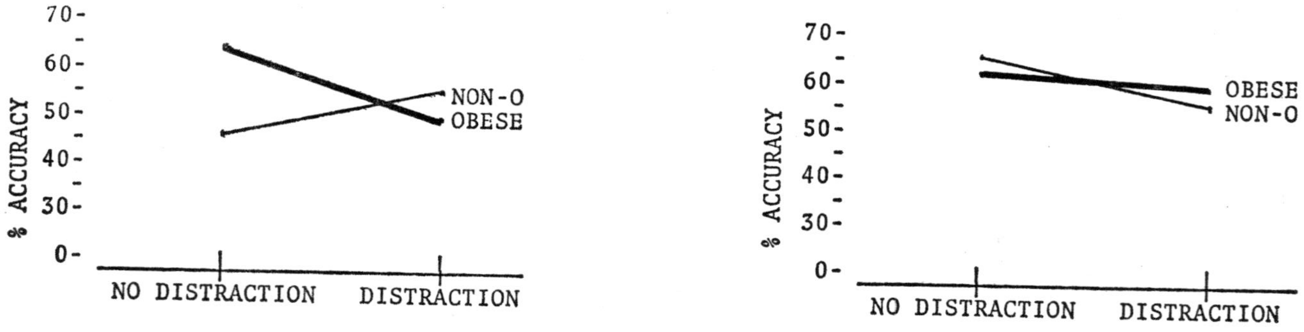

Study I's Proofreading Accuracy

Rodin's (1973) Proofreading Accuracy

tively, $t = 2.42$, $p < .02$, two-tailed). An analysis of performance in the program, at the time of dropping out, indicated that the attrition group reported significantly greater weekly calorie intake ($p < .008$), and significantly fewer calories of expenditure during exercise ($p < .009$) than subjects who remained in treatment. These data suggest that the dropouts had only marginally adhered to the prescribed program and perhaps were insufficiently motivated to follow a rigorous weight reduction regime. Reasons for dropping out given by the 12 subjects contacted included inconvenience (4 subjects), babysitting problems (1 subject), illness (2 subjects), transportation difficulties (1 subject), out-of-state marriage (1 subject), conflicting work schedule (2 subjects), and marital difficulties (1 subject).

Two-way analyses of variance were performed on the pretreatment dependent measures and demographic variables to assess the equivalence of subjects assigned to deposit, no-deposit conditions and to therapist 1 versus therapist 2. Of the 11 analyses, only the socioeconomic levels of the subjects assigned to the two therapists were significantly different ($F = 26.10$, $df = 1,16$, $p < .0005$). Subjects assigned to therapist 1 represented a higher socioeconomic level than subjects assigned to therapist 2 (mean 1.3, 4, respectively). Group differences concerning socioeconomic level would likely have little impact on the dependent measures of weight loss.

General Treatment Effects

The first question dealt with the efficacy of self-management treatment procedures in achieving weight loss, irrespective of the specific assignment to therapist or deposit conditions. Indices of weight loss were obtained from pre- to post-treatment and included pounds lost, reduction index, and change in body density. Correlated t tests of mean group scores indicated that subjects across all conditions exhibited a significant loss of weight as measured by pounds lost (mean = 6.45 pounds, $t = 3.13$, $p < .001$, one-tailed), and reduction index (mean = 16.15, $t = 3.92$, $p < .0008$, one-tailed), and a non-significant increase in residual change scores of body density (mean = .004, $t = 1.45$, $p < .10$, one-tailed). Due to the high variability in the residual change scores of body density,

a non-parametric analysis was also performed. A Wilcoxian test of
signed ranks indicated a significant increase in body density over
the course of treatment ($p < .022$). These data indicate that the
self-management procedures were significantly effective in facilitating weight loss in subjects participating in the treatment
program.

Specific treatment comparisons. The major experimental hypotheses concerned the relative efficacy of deposit versus no-deposit.
If deposit contracts are superior in facilitating weight loss, then
one would predict that subjects in this condition would lose
greater amounts of weight no matter which therapist had seen
them. On the other hand, if subjects seen by one therapist lost
more weight than subjects seen by the second therapist, a significant therapist effect would be indicated. Table 5-3 presents a
2-way (Therapist × Condition) analyses of variance indicating
no significant differences among groups on pounds lost, reduction
index, or change in body density. These data are presented graphically in Figures 5-3 and 5-4. Trends in the reduction index data
suggested that subjects in the deposit group lost somewhat less
weight (non-significant) than subjects in the no-deposit condition
(means = 11.7 and 21.5, respectively) and that subjects seen by
therapist 1 lost less weight (non-significant) than those seen by
therapist 2 (means = 11.2 and 21.0, respectively). These data do
not support the hypotheses that (1) deposit contracts are more
effective in facilitating weight loss in self-management programs,
nor (2) therapist's clinical skill and personal attributes have a
differential effect on weight loss at post treatment beyond the
general skills acquired through a standard therapist training
program.

Maintenance of treatment effects. Data collected on 15 subjects
(out of 20) at two-month follow-up provided the preliminary
assessment of weight maintenance. The relative maintenance of
weight across all subjects was examined with t tests of residual
change scores of weight, reduction index, and body density. These
analyses indicated that all three measures at follow-up were not
significantly different than those at post-treatment. The average
subject regained .45 pounds at follow-up. Supplemental non-
parametric analysis of these data using the Wilcoxin test of signed
ranks further indicated no significant difference from post-treat-

TABLE 5-3

Two-Way Analysis of Variance Using Scheffe's Approximation on Post Residual Change Scores for Reduction Index, Pounds Lost, and Body Density

Source	Reduction Index			Measure Pounds Lost			Body Density		
	df	MS	F	df	MS	F	df	MS	F
Inducement	1	725.0196	2.103	1	21.0103	.2402	1	.00010238	.7262
Therapist	1	803.8571	2.332	1	148.4330	1.6968	1	.00021569	.0000
Inducement X Therapist	1	463.4916	1.344	1	139.1045	1.5901	1	.00006565	.4656
Within Cells	16	344.7514		16	87.47953			.0014097	

Note: N = 20.

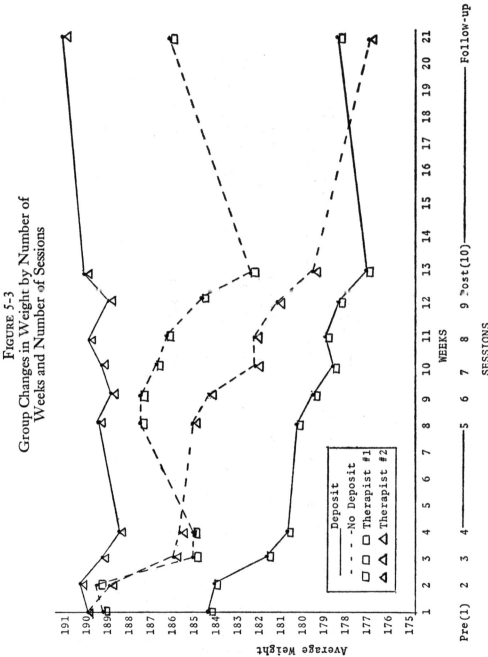

FIGURE 5-3
Group Changes in Weight by Number of
Weeks and Number of Sessions

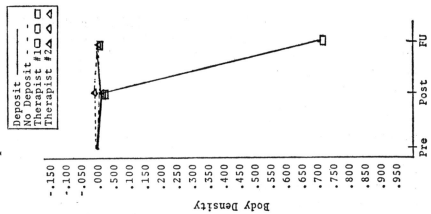

Mean Change in Reduction Index, Pounds Lost, and Body
Density from Treatment to Post-Treatment and Follow-up

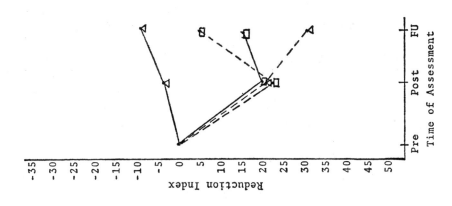

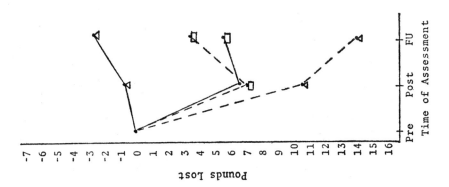

ment to follow-up on weight and reduction index, but that body density had significantly increased ($p < .005$). These findings reflect that weight loss was maintained during follow-up and that body density may have changed in a favorable direction.

It was predicted from the standpoint of attribution theory that subjects who were externally motivated (deposit group) to lose weight would be less inclined to maintain their weight loss than subjects who received no external inducement for weight loss (no-deposit groups). This hypothesis presumed, however, that subjects in these two conditions had perceived their performance to have been influenced by external versus personal factors. A spot check on this assumption obtained at follow-up yielded contradictory evidence. Subjects were correctly able to identify the purpose of the deposit (or absence of a deposit) and they generally indicated that they had accepted the rationale which had been provided. However, when asked whether their weight loss had been attributable to treatment or personal factors, all 10 of the subjects in the deposit condition indicated that their losses had been due to personal factors, whereas four of the subjects in the no-deposit condition felt their progress had been due to personal factors and four felt that treatment factors were the causal agent. A Fisher's exact 2 × 2 test of these data indicated a significant relationship ($p < .027$). It is therefore difficult to ascertain exactly what cognitive attribution sets were operating in these subjects.

Two-way analyses of variance (Therapist × Condition) were also performed to investigate any significant relationship between the independent variables and weight maintenance. Table 5-4 summarizes these data for pounds lost, reduction index, and body density measures, respectively. As can be seen, there was a significant Therapist × Condition interaction for pounds lost ($F = 5.58$, $p < .05$), reduction index ($F = 5.09$, $p < .05$), and a significant main effect for both therapists ($F = 5.57$, $p < .05$) and deposit condition ($F = 5.65$, $p < .05$) on body density measures. Subjects in the deposit condition, across therapists, maintained their weight on a similar level; however, within the no-deposit condition, subjects assigned to therapist 2 lost additional weight between posttreatment and follow-up, while those who had been assigned to therapist 1 regained weight. The significant main effects for thera-

TABLE 5-4

Two-Way Analysis of Variance Using Scheffe's Approximation on Follow-up Residual Change Scores for Reduction Index, Pounds Lost, and Body Density

Source		Reduction Index			Measure Pounds Lost			Body Density	
	df	MS	F	df	MS	F	df	MS	F
Inducement	1	1.1895	.0078	1	6.7724	.7673	1	.387497	5.65*
Therapist	1	595.7490	3.91	1	40.8022	4.62	1	.381685	5.57*
Inducement X Therapist	1	776.2054	5.09*	1	49.2600	5.58*	1	.333514	4.86
Within Cells	11	152.2692		11	8.8258		10**	.068573	

* $p < .05$.
** Body Density obtained on N = 14.

pist and conditions on body density measures indicated that subjects in the deposit condition, compared with those in the no-deposit condition, and subjects assigned to therapist 1, compared with those assigned to therapist 2, increased their body density to a significantly greater degree (see Figure 5-5). The data on weight loss suggest that successful weight maintenance in a sclf-management program may be a combined function of therapist variables and the nature of inducement which was used in the particular treatment program. The somewhat discrepant findings on the body density measure reflect a non-linear relationship between this variable and weight loss, in that subjects assigned to therapist A increased their body density to a significantly greater degree across both conditions, while on weight loss measures in the no-deposit condition, subjects assigned to therapist 1 regained significantly more weight than those assigned to therapist 2. Furthermore, any relationship between weight maintenance and the cognitive attribution set held by subjects remains unclear.

Prediction of Weight Loss

Supplemental correlational analyses were also performed to determine whether successful weight loss during treatment was related to certain demographic and predictive factors. Table 5-5 presents the correlation matrix between the pre-post reduction index and the following scores: no-distraction proofreading accuracy, distraction proofreading accuracy, difference between distraction and no-distraction proofreading accuracy, internal-external locus of control score, extraversion, neuroticism, age, education, socioeconomic level, food calories at end of program, and exercise calories at end of program. These data indicate that except for food calories at end of program, none of these possible predictive and demographic variables are related to reduction index scores. The relationship between food calories at end of program and reduction index suggests that low calorie intake at the end of treatment was associated with successful weight loss. The search for a powerful variable to predict which clients would succeed in a self-management weight loss program emphasizing situational control and a balance between calorie intake and expenditure, was not fruitful.

Figure 5-5
Therapist by Inducement Interactions, to
Post-Treatment and Follow-up

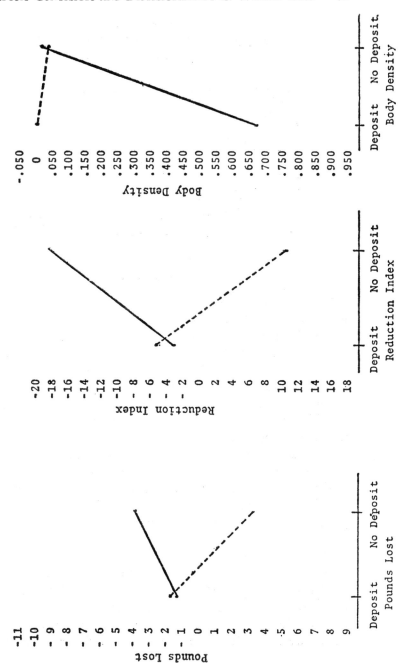

TABLE 5-5
Possible Predictors and Their Correlation
with Reduction Index

Internal-External Locus of Control (Rotter)	+.04
Extraversion (Eysenck)	—.20
Neuroticism (Eysenck)	+.21
Age in Years	+.26
Education in Years	+.24
Socio-Economic Level	+.04
Food Calories at End of Program	—.46*
Exercise Calories at End of Program	—.01
No Distraction % Proofreading Accuracy	—.08
Distraction % Proofreading Accuracy	—.09
Difference % Proofreading Accuracy	—.01

* Significant at the $p < .05$ level two-tailed.

DISCUSSION

The present study has illustrated that once again self-management procedures were effective in reduction and maintenance of weight, that stimulus boundedness as measured by distractibility in Rodin's (1973) proofreading task was not a valid predictor of weight loss, that deposit contracts were not demonstrably superior to no-deposit in achieving weight loss, and that weight maintenance was due to a complex interaction of both therapist variables and the nature of inducement used in the particular treatment program.

The failure to find a significant relationship between distractibility and weight loss is perhaps due to the non-replication of Rodin's original findings and the possiblity that a valid measure of stimulus boundedness was not obtained. The fact that the present replication was based upon an older, female sample recruited from the community, instead of upon college males, may explain the discrepancy in findings. Alternatively, the measure of stimulus boundedness to food related cues, as opposed to non-food cues, may prove to be a more powerful predictor variable of performance in a clinical program directly concerned with consumption of food. In any event, the present study did not constitute a conclusive test of the possible relationship between responsiveness to external cues and performance in a self-management weight reduction program.

The findings concerning the efficacy of self-management procedures are similar to those of Mahoney (1974) who found that emphasis on habit change as opposed to weight loss per se is an effective treatment strategy to achieve both weight reduction and maintenance. The failure to find a differential effect of deposit contracts differs somewhat from findings by Jeffrey (1974) and Abrahms and Allen (1974). However, in the present study, the inclusion of a no-deposit group in addition to a deposit group wherein all money was returned at the end of treatment allowed for a more definitive test of the efficacy of monetary inducements and their effect on weight maintenance. The factorial representation of therapists in the experimental design eliminated the potential confounding of treatment effects by the factors of therapist's skill and personal attributes. The significant Therapist × Condition interaction obtained at follow-up suggests that, under the deposit condition, therapist factors played no differential role in treatment efficacy, but when the external leverage of deposits was not employed, one therapist was significantly more effective than the other in facilitating weight maintenance. While the possibility of systematic differences in group composition cannot be ruled out, these findings highlight the need for more thorough investigation of therapist factors in relation to the effectiveness of self-management treatment procedures.

Attrition. The substantial attrition rate (41 percent) encountered in this study highlights an important problem encountered in the treatment of obesity. Unlike some investigations, no penalty was placed upon termination of treatment in either condition, and consequently it was relatively easy for subjects to drop out of treatment. As a group, these subjects differed from those who remained in treatment only in their level of education. Close inspection of their performance prior to dropping out allowed identification of several characteristics common to subjects in the attrition group. Compared with those subjects who remained in treatment, dropouts exercised significantly less and consumed significantly more calories of food. The homogeneity in variance of these scores was highly significant ($p < .009$). Despite the reasons they gave for dropping out, these data suggest that subjects who terminated treatment prematurely were not strictly adhering to the rules of the treatment program. Whether thorough screening on motivational factors would have excluded these subjects from the treatment program is open to question, but in the early stages of treatment, dropouts appeared less committed to a weight reduction program than those subjects who eventually completed treatment.

Differential Effectiveness

As with previous research on self-management programs, high variability in treatment response was found in the present study. Based upon both clinical and objective data, three hypotheses may be generated to account for this finding: 1) as with dropouts, subjects who make little progress in this type of self-management program may actually have been poorly motivated for behavior change and included in the treatment sample due to a faulty screening process. In the present study, far more attention was placed upon the specified demographic, availability, and other screening criteria to the possible expense of the more intangible motivational criteria. The implication of this observation for future investigations is to make provisions for a thorough evaluation of the subject's personal commitment to weight loss and motivation to make significant changes in life style to accommodate this goal; 2) previous experience with other professionals or weight reduction clubs were reported by 85 percent of the subjects in this sample. It is likely that this previous experience may have engendered in many subjects a set of preconceived treatment expectations that were dissonant with the aims of the present program. This presumption calls for a thorough orientation at the beginning stages of treatment to offset any previous learning in a weight reduction context which would be counterproductive to a self-management regime; 3) high variability in weight loss within treatment groups is also a function of subjects who overzealously lose far more than the desired 1-2 pounds per week. For example, in the present study, one subject (D.W.) lost 41¼ pounds over the 13-week program, an average of 3.2 pounds per week. It is quite reasonable to expect that this subject, and those like her, deviated from the program in perhaps several ways to achieve such substantial weight loss. The overzealous subject, who is perhaps as much a treatment failure as the subject who resists dietary and exercise modification, may be subtly reinforced by investigators whose payoffs come from impressive outcome data. Unfortunately, the subtle encouragement of drastic weight loss measures is not compatible with the long-range treatment goals of teaching clients habit changes which may be continued through life.

Additional suggestions may be delineated which would undoubtedly contribute to maximal effectiveness in self-management weight loss programs. Individualization of the treatment program to conform to the client's particular life pattern, personality, and eating habits may be a preferable alternative to the standardized regime used in most treatment studies. Unfortunately, individualized treatment programs may reduce the comparability of subjects and treatments for research purposes, but increases in effectiveness may be well worth the price. More attention may be paid to therapist factors in order to help persuade commitment to the program and deal with certain forms of client resistance. Investigation of therapist status variables, such as age, professional background, and perceived professional competence may identify an important variable to facilitate weight loss. The use of former obese clients as therapists may also prove to be one effective alternative to enhance the therapist's credibility. When self-management procedures are used in a group context, attention should also be directed to group composition. Peer reinforcement and support accompanied by task-directed group goals may be highly effective in facilitating consistent weight loss and habit change among all group members.

Maintenance of Treatment Effects

The findings that therapists were differentially effective at follow-up depending upon whether deposit contracts were used or not underscores the need to identify which treatment variations are most effective with which therapists. These suggestive findings concerning the Therapist × Inducement condition interactions must be interpreted in light of potential intrasession history effects and subsequent confounding of the particular group composition with therapist effects.

The somewhat discrepant findings between weight loss and body density measures suggest that more research is needed to understand the properties of density measures and their relationship to reduction in weight. Interpretation of maintenance effects based upon the weight loss measures suggests that deposit contracts may be useful in that they tend to obviate the need for less obvious forms of clinical skill to facilitate subject performance. It should be remembered that the group that continued to lose weight at follow-up and, conversely, the group which regained the most weight had both participated in the no-deposit condition. Although subjects motivated through use of deposits were more consistent in their maintenance of weight loss across therapists, both the best and the worst weight maintenance were found in subjects receiving no external inducement. Thus, when no external incentive was used, therapist factors appeared to play a crucial role in whether the subjects progressed or not.

In addition to the possible role of the therapist, numerous other factors may be isolated to insure maintenance of weight loss. Amplifying upon those outlined by Abrahms and Allen (1974), these include: 1) Stimulus control exercises, dietary restrictions, and exercise programs should be prescribed which may be realistically followed indefinitely without inducing boredom, nutritional imbalances, or undue inconvenience. Gimmicks should be avoided which, although effective on a short-term basis, may be difficult to follow for extended periods of time. 2) Emphasis should be placed on eating habit change, and not weight loss. In line with Mahoney's (1974) findings, focusing clients on actual eating habit change is likely to have more lasting effects than emphasizing weight loss per se. 3) The social environment should be reprogrammed to elicit cooperation from spouses, family, and friends. If one adopts the notion that obesity is under the control of situational factors, the reinforcing or punishing consequences from significant others constitute a critical contextual ingredient. Reprogramming the social environment may also be necessary in effecting changes in life style. Families may be encouraged to pursue new social contacts which would be supportive of treatment goals and recreational activities which do not rely heavily on consumatory behavior (e.g., joining a bicycle club instead of a gourmet club). 4) Attention should also be paid to phasing out therapeutic involvement. Trial maintenance periods and booster sessions are examples of phase-out procedures which may help insure maintenance of treatment effects. Upon completion of a treatment program, clients should also be encouraged to adopt a contingency plan for when weight exceeds a critical value. If obesity is construed as a lifelong struggle, it is perhaps appropriate to consider a lifelong treatment involvement with a self-management consultant much like periodic visits to one's doctor or dentist. Problems with maintenance may actually result from the faulty assumption by professionals that well-rooted patterns of behavior are permanently amenable to change through a few hours of professional contact extending over several weeks time.

ACKNOWLEDGMENT

This study was based partially upon Master's theses by Ronald Nathan and Lois Schiavo under the direction of John P. Vincent. Gratitude is expressed to Bruce Graunke and Jim Breckenridge, who faithfully served as therapists, and to Ed Charlesworth and Aileen McMurrer who more than just assisted in the completion of this project. Thanks also to Louis Schiavo and Linzy Messerly, our computer consultants.

Chapter 6

A Proposal for a Macro Environmental Analysis in the Prevention and Treatment of Obesity

D. Balfour Jeffrey

Obesity results from either an excessive intake of calories and/ or insufficient energy expenditure. The causes of this imbalance are not entirely clear. There are a few known medical disorders such as Cushing's syndrome which cause obesity (Williams, 1968). However, there seems to be growing consensus that most cases of obesity result from environmental factors and *not* medical factors (Mayer, 1968; Stuart and Davis, 1972).

An analysis of these environmental factors can occur at two levels—micro and macro. A micro analysis focuses on the eating, exercise, and psychological patterns of the individual. Most behavioral and traditional research (e.g., Abramson, 1973; Bruch, 1943; Jeffrey, in press, b; Jeffrey and Katz, in press; Stunkard and Mahoney, in press) has focused on treating individual, obese patients. This micro research is continuing to add to the understanding and treatment of obesity.

The other level of work consists of a macro analysis. This focuses on the total society and how the society facilitates or impedes good eating habits, physical activity habits, and weight management. While there are millions of people who are starving in other parts of the world, the United States is one of the few nations that has a major problem with obesity. Obesity in Amer-

98

ica, in part, is related to the affluence of our society, the availability of food, particularly junk food (i.e., food high in sugar and low in nutrients), the mechanization of our society, and the decrease of physical activity (Mayer, 1968; Stuart and Davis, 1972). Furthermore, there is growing recognition of the profound influence of advertising in conditioning our food preferences and consumption of non-nutritional, high calorie foods such as sugar-coated cereals, candies, soft drinks, and beer (Gussow, 1972).

The problem of obesity is not one of not knowing what to do; medically, we know what we should do. Physicians and nutritionists know what foods we should be eating. Physicians and physical therapists know what physical activity we should be engaging in. The problem is getting society at large and people individually to change their eating and physical activity habits. This is a behavioral problem, *not* a medical problem.

At a societal level, the question is how do we increase good eating and physical activity habits? Or conversely, how do we decrease bad eating and physical activity habits? What do we know about learning principles and behavior modification that we can apply at a societal level?

Before proceeding any further, let us make an assumption, for the sake of this discussion, that our political leaders and the public said to the behaviorists, "Here is a mandate to improve our eating patterns, physical activity, and weight management. Do whatever you need to do." Let us assume that mandate was given for the ensuing part of this discussion. Following are a number of proposals which are designed to modify the eating habits and physical activity habits of millions of people at a societal level. These proposals are by no means comprehensive, nor are they without their difficulties, but hopefully they will stimulate us to start thinking of behavior modification programs at this level of analysis and intervention.

PROPOSALS FOR INCREASING GOOD EATING BEHAVIORS

Improved Nutrition Education

We need to improve the dissemination of information about good nutrition, eating habits, and weight control to health professionals, elementary and secondary school teachers, and the public at large. For example, Emory University Medical School instituted an interdisciplinary committee on nutrition. The committee has recognized that physicians, nurses, and other health professionals receive little formal education in nutrition; consequently, they have developed a new nutrition curriculum for physicians, nurses, and other health professionals in order to improve their training in this area. Health educators are also recognizing that at the elementary and secondary school level there is a need for a more informative and interesting nutrition curriculum. Finally, there is also a need to educate the general public. For example, the American Dietetic Association, in conjunction with other agencies, sponsors a National Good Nutrition Week. This week is designed to make the public more aware of the relationship between good nutrition and good health.

Improved Food Labeling

Clear, concise, and informative labeling of all foods is desirable so that American consumers will be able to identify and purchase nutritious, low calorie foods. New food labeling regulations by the Food and Drug Administration have been instituted in the last few years. Charles Edwards, Commissioner of the Food and Drug Administration, said, "These regulations will bring about the most significant change in food labeling since food labeling began" (U.S. Department of Health, Education, and Welfare, 1973). Hopefully, this information will assist individuals in buying nutritious, low calorie foods. The new nutrition labeling act, effective 1975, requires the following nutrition information per serving: serving size, servings per container, calories, protein, carbohydrates, fat, and percentage of U.S. Recommended Daily Allowances. The caloric content of the food is included, thus conveniently providing information for the person who is trying to lose weight. These new regulations are an important step toward improving nutrition and weight management. However, the nutrition labeling is voluntary for most foods. Only if a food has a nutrient added to it or if a nutritional claim is made for the food must the food include "nutrition information per serving."

What about the caloric content of cookies, candy bars, ice cream, beer, or soft drinks? The consumer is still not told how many calories are in these foods. It seems reasonable and simple to extend the Food and Drug Administration's food labeling regulation to include *all* foods. The consumer would then at last have sufficient information to buy nutritious, low calorie foods.

Examine the Role of Vending Machines on the
Consumption of Food

There is an increasing amount of food sold from vending machines. Although there is nothing wrong with food sold from vending machines, what concerns a growing number of health professionals is that most of these foods are "junk" foods. Often you cannot buy nutritious, low calorie foods even if you want to, because these foods are not stocked in vending machines. Recently, a few educational institutions have examined the influence of vending machines on their students.

The Dallas School Board (1975) was concerned with this issue and on January 22, 1975, passed the following regulation:

> The Board of Education believes that a student has the right to high quality of nutrition and excellent health education. Vending machines in schools shall offer optimal choices to students and all foods and drinks sold in vending machines shall be nutritious and selected for maximal appeal to students, excluding any foods or drinks with a highly concentrated sugar base. Accessibility to vending machines shall be controlled and shall not compete with regular school lunch program and instruction. . . . Machines shall be stocked with such items as fruit and vegetable juices, dietary soft drinks, milk, nuts, seeds, cheese products, crackers, fresh fruits, chips, etc.

This proposal is innovative and should be seriously considered for adoption in school districts throughout our nation. These regulations would, if implemented, provide children with opportunities for purchasing nutritious, low calorie foods, and for developing good eating habits.

Recently, Jean Mayer, a noted nutritionist, and a number of other people concerned with nutrition proposed to the Federal Government that it has a responsibility for the good health of its workers and citizens. They proposed that 50 percent of all foods sold in vending machines on government property be nutritious, low calorie foods. Adults would then at least have some choice in what they purchase and eat, a choice they often do *not* now have.

Examine the Role of Advertising in the Conditioning of Our Food Preferences and Consumption

Over 700 million dollars was spent in our country in 1973 on food and beverage advertisement (U.S. Department of Commerce, 1973). That money would not be spent if it did not modify and control our eating and drinking behaviors. Recent studies have examined the influence of food advertisement on children (Gussow, 1972). It has been found that 60-80 percent of all children's commercials are for food, drink, and vitamin ads (Choate, 1971).

Television in the United States is regulated, in part, by the Federal Government, which controls the licensing of stations and what can be advertised. The selling of hard liquor on television has always been banned. The growing concern about cigarette smoking and lung cancer prompted a regulation which required an anti-smoking commercial for so many pro-smoking commercials. Then Congress went even further and prohibited any advertisement for cigarettes on television or radio (U.S. Public Law 91-222).

Since food advertising has a profound influence on children's buying and eating habits, we might consider regulating the type and quantity of food advertisements on children's television programs. We might consider that every time there is an advertisement for a junk food, an anti-junk food commercial or one nutritious food commercial would be required. We might even consider banning the advertisement of all junk foods on television.

Investigate the Role of Subsidies and Taxes on Our Food Buying and Consumption

The Department of Agriculture subsidizes the growing of a variety of crops. One of the crops subsidized is tobacco. The American Medical Association is now lobbying with other health associations to eliminate all farm subsidies for tobacco. They argue that since we have established a causal relationship between cigarette smoking and cancer, it does not make good health or financial sense for the Department of Health, Education, and Welfare to spend millions of dollars each year trying to reduce cigarette smoking, while the Department of Agriculture subsidizes the growing of tobacco.

These recommendations might be extended so that the Department of Agriculture would not provide subsidies for any crop which has some health hazards associated with that crop. Some health professionals have concluded that our increasing consumption of sugar is a health hazard because it adds high calories with few nutrients, increases dental problems, and takes money which could be spent for more nutritious foods (American Dental Association, 1961; Burkett, 1973). Therefore, it might be in the nation's health interest not to provide farm subsidies to grow sugar.*

We also might examine the role of taxes in modifying our purchasing and eating behavior. Our society has always used taxes on specific products to generate income and to reduce the purchase of those products that society has deemed unhealthy. For example, the large tax on cigarettes is used to generate income for education and health projects, and, hopefully, to discourage cigarette buying. There is also a tax on liquor for similar reasons. There also might be a tax on sugar or a tax on vending machines selling junk foods in order to increase their price and, therefore, decrease somewhat the consumption of these foods; as a byproduct, tax revenue would be generated for health programs.

In summary, these proposals are presented to increase good eating habits and decrease our bad eating habits. The same kind of approach could be attempted to increase our good physical activity behaviors and decrease poor physical activity behaviors.

PROPOSALS FOR INCREASING GOOD PHYSICAL ACTIVITY HABITS

Improved Education

Physical education programs similar to the proposed nutrition education programs need to be increased and upgraded for health

---

*Farmers do not need to worry whether they might go out of business, for there are many other food crops that can be grown in place of sugar. Furthermore, with today's food shortages, more nutritious crops such as wheat or soybeans are needed to help feed the many hungry people of the world.

professionals, students, and the public. On the public level, we already have the President's Council on Physical Fitness which sponsors physical fitness advertisements on television as well as other physical activity programs. Physical education programs at all levels should be expanded.

Establish National Standards for Sports and Recreation Facilities

A comprehensive study might be undertaken to establish minimal national standards for the type and number of sports and recreational facilities needed per 10,000 people. These plans should obviously consider the convenience and access to these facilities so people will be inclined to use them. After the comprehensive study is completed, efforts should be directed at implementing the national standards by Federal, state, and local funding to build and maintain these sports and recreational facilities.

Employer Sponsored Sports Facilities

Most grade schools, high schools, and colleges provide sports facilities, programs, and incentives for their students or employees to use while attending school or while "on the job." A few governmental, medical, and corporate institutions provide employees with similar physical activity facilities and programs. For example, the U.S. Department of Justice in Washington has a gym and an active exercise program for its employees. Grady Hospital of Emory University has now started a limited exercise program for the house staff two days a week. The Phillips Oil Company has a very active sports and exercise program for its employees (Heuston, 1973). Phillips provides a wide variety of gym facilities, sports programs, and awards for participation in these programs. One often sees before work, at lunch, or after work, people going to the gym and having an exercise break rather than a food break. These fine examples of employers' efforts to maintain good health and weight control of their employees through sound physical fitness are, unfortunately, the exception rather than the rule. Hopefully, more institutions will develop similar programs.

Taxes and Physical Activity

Today there is an energy crisis, particularly a shortage of oil. In examining the energy crunch, there really is a large source of energy that is untapped in our society—the adipose tissue of millions of Americans. There are approximately 70,000,000 Americans who are overweight, and if we assume that they average 10 pounds overweight (a conservative estimate), that is equal to 700,000,000 pounds of fat, multiplied by 3,500 calories per pound, or over 2,450,000,000,000 calories of energy stored in the fat cells of Americans. How can we use this energy source and save our precious gasoline? The State of Oregon is already indirectly solving, in part, this problem. They allocate 1 percent of their gasoline taxes for building bike paths that are safe and convenient. In increasing bicycling, both for recreation *and* for transportation, we will burn off fat, reduce our weight, release tension, decrease appetites, improve our cardiovascular conditioning, decrease air pollution, and reduce gasoline consumption.

In summary, a number of proposals have been presented for modifying the eating and physical activity habits of individuals and society in general. These proposals are neither comprehensive nor exhaustive. Obviously, other proposals can be and should be made. My hope is to get myself, you, and others to start thinking of the possibilities of a macro environmental analysis of the causes, preventions, and treatments of obesity at the societal level.

These proposals are based on the assumption that there is a mandate from our political leaders and the public to improve our eating habits, physical activity habits, and weight management. That mandate does not exist at the present time. Since these proposals really involve the political processes of our country, implementing these proposals will involve influencing the behaviors of our political leaders and the public. As concerned citizens, parents, and professionals, we have a responsibility to encourage our professional associations, political leaders, and the general public to support effective nutrition, physical activity, and weight control programs.

Part III

MEDICAL AND NUTRITIONAL ISSUES AND TECHNIQUES

INTRODUCTION

The chapters in Part III provide information on the relationship of obesity to other cardiovascular risk factors (particularly elevated blood pressure, elevated levels of serum cholesterol and triglycerides, and diabetes), discuss the importance of good nutrition during weight loss programs, and present an example of a behaviorally based training program for nutrition educators following the Keller method.

Antonio M. Gotto, Jr., John P. Foreyt, and Lynne W. Scott, in Chapter 7, "Cardiovascular risk factors," not only discuss the medical importance of weight control for reducing the risks of cardiovascular complications but also stress the need for individuals and families to adopt an eating plan low in cholesterol and saturated fats. They provide a concise and detailed discussion of the hyperlipidemia and the dietary factors which affect the level of cholesterol in the blood.

In Chapter 8, "Nutrition during weight loss," Lynne W. Scott, John P. Foreyt, and Antonio M. Gotto, Jr., discuss some of the characteristics of the successful dieter and provide guidelines for planning diets aimed at weight loss. The authors make a strong argument for the behavioral therapist to be well versed in the basic principles of nutrition, and they emphasize the importance of the behavioral therapist-nutritionist team working to-gether when planning and conducting weight loss programs. They describe the HELP Your Heart Eating Plan, a diet which can be individualized to meet the eating habits of obese persons and is flexible enough to accommodate different lifestyles without drastic alterations in types of food eaten. The basic principles of the plan include a decrease in cholesterol intake, decrease in level of saturated fat intake, and an increase in the level of polyunsat-urated fat.

Valerie B. Knotts, in Chapter 9, "Training nutrition educators: Behavior modification in the kitchen," describes for nutrition educators one example of how to set up a course in dietary man-agement. She also provides examples of projects that her students carried out using the principles learned in her course.

Chapter 7

Cardiovascular Risk Factors

Antonio M. Gotto, Jr., John P. Foreyt
and Lynne W. Scott

About three-quarters of all people who die or are disabled by cardiovascular diseases have one or more of the three major risk factors: elevation of serum cholesterol, elevation of blood pressure, and cigarette smoking (Task Force on Atherosclerosis of the National Heart and Lung Institute, 1971). In addition to these three, there are several secondary risk factors: obesity, elevation of serum triglycerides, heredity, diabetes, high saturated fat diet, lack of physical activity, and personality type A (i.e., a striving, aggressive, impatient, pressured individual).

Obesity directly or indirectly relates to a number of these factors. It tends to make hypertension worse for someone with a tendency toward hypertension. It exacerbates an elevation in serum triglycerides, if there is a propensity for this problem. It makes diabetes worse, is related to a lack of physical activity, and may be related to a high saturated fat diet and to personality type.

ATHEROSCLEROSIS

The underlying cause of most cardiovascular disease is a pathological process known as atherosclerosis. Atherosclerosis probably begins early in life.

This work was supported by Grant No. HL 17269 from the National Heart and Lung Institute for the National Research and Demonstration Center.

109

FIGURE 7-1

Cross Section Drawing of an Artery

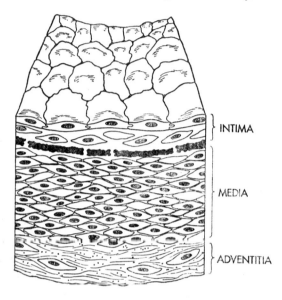

INTIMA

MEDIA

ADVENTITIA

FIGURE 7-2

Atherosclerosis is characterized by a deposit of fatty substances in the intimal layer resulting in reduction of the blood flow through the lumen of the artery. Cross section of normal artery is at left; longitudinal section shows increasing atherosclerosis from left to right; cross section of atherosclerotic artery is on right.

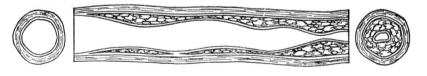

Figure 7-1 represents an artery. The innermost part of the artery, the intima, is only one cell in thickness at birth. Arthero-sclerosis is characterized by a deposit of fatty substances in this intimal layer. This can result in a reduction in the blood flow through the lumen of the artery (Figure 7-2). Cholesterol and its chemical esters are the major fatty or lipid substances accumulating within the intima. The cholesterol that is deposited comes primarily from the bloodstream and is derived both from the individual's diet and from endogenous synthesis, being made both in the liver and in the gut. The higher the level of cholesterol in the blood, the greater the tendency to deposit cholesterol in the wall of the artery. Other fats, such as phospholipids, are synthesized within the arterial wall and accumulate there along with the cholesterol. If the narrowing of the artery becomes severe enough, there may be an insufficient amount of blood flow so that at times of stress there wil be inadequate blood and oxygen carried to the tissue or organ to allow it to carry on its normal activities. Chest pain, or angina pectoris, one of the clinical symptoms of coronary heart disease, may result from involvement of one or more coronary arteries.

The manifestations of arteriosclerosis depend upon which arterial bed or beds are primarily affected. If the arteries supplying the brain are involved, then the manifestations may be cerebrovascular insufficiency. The consequence may be a cerebrovascular acident or a stroke. If the coronary arteries are affected, the manifestations may be angina pectoris, sudden death, a coronary thrombosis, or myocardial infarction, i.e., a heart attack. When an artery carrying blood to the heart is sufficiently damaged a blood clot may form, the part of the heart that derives its blood supply from that particular artery will die. If it is the artery carrying blood to the kidneys or to the extremities that is affected, hypertension or cramps or pains in the legs when walking may occur.

What is the relationship between arteriosclerosis, diet, serum lipids and obesity? Let us take the example of an inherited type of high blood cholesterol, familial hypercholesterolemia, or Type II hyperlipidemia (Fredrickson and Levy, 1972; Goldstein, Dana, Brunschede, and Brown, 1975; Goldstein, Hazzard, Schrott, and Bierman, 1973; Goldstein, Schrott, Hazzard, Bierman, and Motulsky, 1973. For males with this disorder, the incidence of heart attacks and coronary deaths is alarmingly high (Table 7-1) (Slack, 1969). The female is protected by about 10-15 years, compared with the male. We do not know the reason for this but suspect that it is related in part to the female sex hormones.

The Framingham Study (Dawber, Kannel, Revotskie and Kagan, 1962) showed that there was a strong relationship be-

Table 7-1

Affected First Degree Relatives of Patients with Familial
Type II Hyperlipidemia or Hypercholesterolemia*

MALES			FEMALES		
AGE	ISCHEMIC HEART DISEASE*		AGE	ISCHEMIC HEART DISEASE*	
	% INCIDENCE	% DEATHS		% INCIDENCE	% DEATHS·
30-39	28.2	15.4	30-39	0	0
40-49	62.8	38.4	40-49	6.1	· 0
50-59	89.4	. 73.6	50-59	46.1	14.2
60-69	100.0	86.8	60-69·	70.1	14.2
Mean age of onset = 43.8 years IHD			Mean age of onset = 57.1 years IHD		

* This table is used with the permission of *The Lancet* and Dr. Joan Slack.

tween angina pectoris, sudden death, or myocardial infarction and increases in body weight. The correlation was stronger for men than for women. There was also a positive correlation between crude morbidity ratios and relative weight.

PLASMA LIPID TRANSPORT, THE PLASMA LIPOPROTEINS AND HYPERLIPIDEMIA

The two main fatty substances in the blood with which the physician is concerned are cholesterol and triglyceride. If either one or both of these are elevated, we refer to the condition as hyperlipidemia. The body has evolved a way of using protein and phospholipid substances as detergents to keep the neutral lipids, the cholesterol and triglyceride, in solution as they are transported in the body. The mechanism of lipid transport involves a series of complexes known as lipoproteins (i.e., the complex consists of lipids and proteins) (Table 7-2). If the elevation of triglyceride or cholesterol is defined in terms of which specific family or class of lipoproteins in the blood is abnormal, then we refer to the

TABLE 7-2

HUMAN PLASMA LIPOPROTEINS

FAMILY	CHYLOMICRONS	VLDL	LDL	HDL
Density Range	<1.006	<1.006	1.019 - 1.063	1.063 - 1.210
Major Lipids	Exogenous Triglycerides	Endogenous Triglycerides	Cholesterol Cholesteryl Esters	Phospholipid Cholesteryl Esters
% Protein	2	10	25	50

TABLE 7-3

Magnitude of Major Fat Transport Tasks in Plasma

Lipid	Lipoprotein or Carrier	Grams/Day
Free fatty acids	Albumin	50-150
Triglycerides		
Exogenous	Chylomicrons	70-150
Endogenous	VLDL	25- 50
Cholesterol	Chylomicrons, VLDL, LDL, HDL	1

condition using the more specific term, hyperlipoproteinemia. These disorders may be primary, they may be inherited, or they may be secondary to some other disorder, such as pancreatitis, hypothyroidism, diabetes mellitus, kidney disease or liver disease (Fredrickson and Levy, 1972).

The quantities of the plasma fats transported each day and the lipoprotein carriers responsible are given in Table 7-3. Most of the energy to support minute-to-minute activities comes from the oxidation of unesterified fatty acids. These are carried primarily in association with albumin. When the body needs energy, an epinephrine-sensitive lipase enzyme is activated and leads to a breakdown or hydrolysis of triglyceride at adipose tissue sites, releasing unesterified fatty acids into the bloodstream. An intracellular hormone-sensitive lipase regulates this process; it is activated by cyclic AMP. The fatty acids are then carried to the body and supply its energy needs. The excess fatty acids over and above the body's requirements are taken up by the liver where they are reincorporated into triglyceride. They are then secreted back into the bloodstream as very low density lipoproteins (VLDL). Most of the triglyceride produced by the body is made this way. In contrast to the rapid turnover and metabolism of the unesterified fatty acids and triglycerides, the cholesterol in the body shows only a very slow turnover. For this reason, if the body is in a positive state of balance with respect to cholesterol and accumulates a small amount each day, significant quantities of cholesterol can accumulate within the body tissues and eventually lead to the production of atherosclerosis.

There are four different families of the lipoprotein substances in the blood (Table 7-2) (Fredrickson, Levy and Lees, 1967). The largest of these, the chylomicrons, carries most of the triglyceride that comes from the diet (the exogenous triglyceride) (Figures 7-3, 7-4). Cholesterol, triglyceride, and phospholipids are contained in the food substances in the intestine. These are broken down by enzymes in the small bowel and the triglyceride is resynthesized in the wall of the intestine. The fatty acids containing less than 12 carbon atoms go directly into the portal blood. The longer chain fatty acids are used to resynthesize the triglyceride, which are incorporated into the chylomicron lipoprotein particle and are transported in the lymph to the circulation. As these large particles pass through the peripheral tissues, the triglycerides are broken down by an enzyme called lipoprotein lipase. The partially degraded particles are called remnants (Redgrave, 1969; Stein, Stein, Goodman and Fidge, 1969). They have become triglyceride-poor and relatively cholesterol-enriched. They are transported back to the liver where they are taken up and further catabolized. The VLDL or pre-β-lipoproteins carry most of the triglyceride made in the liver. Most of the cholesterol and cholesteryl esters that are carried in the bloodstream are transported by the low density lipoproteins (LDL) or β-lipoproteins. The high density lipoproteins (HDL) or α-lipoproteins are probably less affected by diet than the other families. HDL tend to be higher in females than in males, perhaps due to differences in the estrogenic female sex hormones. HDL may scavenge cholesterol from the

FIGURE 7-3

Metabolism of chylomicrons in the body. They are made in the intestine and carry mainly dietary triglyceride. Please see text for further description

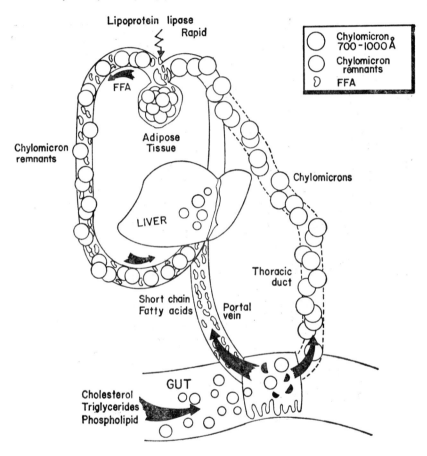

tissues and play some protective role against the development of arteriosclerosis (Stein and Stein, 1973).

Dietary influences on the plasma lipoproteins are complex and differ for each family. But in less than 12 hours after a fatty meal, the presence of chylomicrons is not unusual and causes turbidity of plasma or serum.

If a subject has a tendency toward high levels of VLDL in the

FIGURE 7-4

Metabolism of VLDL in the body. They are made in the liver and to a lesser
extent in the intestine. Please see text for further description

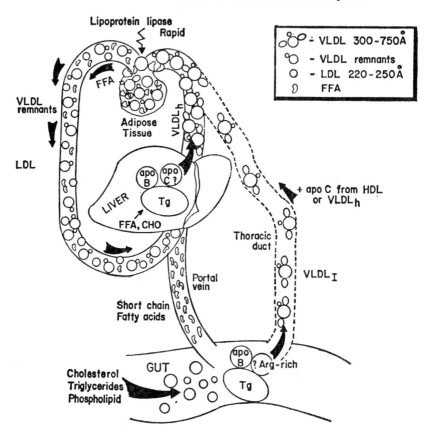

blood, this problem is exacerbated by an excess in calories of alcohol, and, in some individuals, of simple sugars such as sucrose.
Any condition that increases the amount of FFA circulating to
the liver will tend to enhance hepatic triglyceride and VLDL synthesis. The chylomicrons reflect the exogenous fat in the diet;
while the VLDL depend upon the balance of calories, the consumption of alcohol and in some instances the proportion of
calories in simple sugars.

As VLDL circulate through the peripheral tissues, it is thought that they are either catabolized to LDL or are converted to remnant particles and further metabolized by the liver, analogous to the processes described above for chylomicrons. There are many investigators who believe that the remnant particles, representing partially degraded lipoproteins, may be taken up by the arterial wall and contribute to the development of arteriosclerosis.

The LDL, which transport one-half to two-thirds of the total cholesterol in the plasma are decreased by the amount of saturated or animal fat in the diet and by the total quantity of dietary cholesterol (Keys, Anderson, and Grande, 1965). The ratio of polyunsaturated to saturated fat is only about 0.3 in the average American diet. It should be increased to about 1 in order to achieve a 10% reduction in serum cholesterol. In effectiveness in lowering the cholesterol concentration, adding 2 gms of polyunsaturated fat is approximately equivalent to removing 1 gm. of saturated fat from the diet.

OBESITY AND LIPOPROTEIN METABOLISM

The relationships between obesity and lipoprotein metabolism are complex (Vague and Vague, 1974). As far as triglycerides are concerned, a caloric excess and an increased flow of FFA to the liver leads to an overproduction of VLDL and to endogenous hypertriglyceridemia. Under these circumstances, the clearance of chylomicrons, representing exogenous triglyceride, may also be impaired, possibly due to a common pathway for the catabolism of VLDL and chylomicrons (Brunzell, Hazzard, Porte, and Bierman, 1973). In contrast to hypertriglyceridemia, hypercholesterolemia does not correlate well with the degree of obesity. It is thought that there is an oversynthesis of cholesterol in obese subjects, primarily in adipose tissue (Miettinen, 1974). This tissue cholesterol does not cause a significant increase in the cholesterol level in the blood or the plasma. Presumably, the excess cholesterol is either stored in the tissue or is transported back to the liver where it may be excreted into the bile and stool as either neutral sterol, i.e., cholesterol, or as bile acids. The body cannot completely break down cholesterol, but can convert it to bile acids. In the obese person, although there is an oversynthesis of cholesterol, there is also an increase in sterol turnover or cholesterol turnover so that more cholesterol and more bile acids are excreted in the stool or a greater tissue storage of cholesterol occurs. If the cholesterol appeared in the bloodstream, obesity would probably have even much greater consequences on the development of arteriosclerosis. The mechanism whereby obesity increases cholesterol synthesis is not known but may be related to overeating.

ETIOLOGY OF OBESITY

Let us turn to obesity in man and ask some questions concerning its etiology, which may begin early in life. Perhaps the most fundamental question is can we modify the number of adipose cells? Much of the research in this area has been done by Jules Hirsch and his associates (Hirsch, 1971, 1972; Hirsch and Han, 1969; Hirsch, Knittle and Salans, 1966) at Rockefeller University. For the rat, the ultimate number of adipocytes can be decreased by underfeeding the very young animal. In man, the answer to this question is not known. Most obese individuals have some increase in adipocyte size; yet, in nearly all cases, particularly when the obesity is of juvenile onset, there is a striking increase in the *number* of adipocytes. Decreasing the number of adipocytes by underfeeding early in life of subjects susceptible to developing obesity seems a more logical approach than waiting until the excess number of adipocytes has already been achieved. An average non-obese person has 25 to 30 x 10^9 adipocytes. With obesity, this number increases 3 to 5 times. The periods when most adipose cells are laid down are thought to be late in gestation, in the first year of life, and in early adolescence. These probably are critical times when it is important to control the development of obesity; if obesity occurs at such times it may be accompanied by an excessive increase in the number of adipocytes.

METABOLIC EFFECTS OF SPONTANEOUS OBESITY

What are the metabolic effects of spontaneous obesity and can these be directly related to or separated from the amount of carbohydrate in the diet? (Sims, Bray, Danforth, Glennon, Horton, Salans and O'Connell, 1974). One of the effects of obesity is an

TABLE 7-4

Metabolic Effects of
Spontaneous Obesity

1. Plasma insulin ↑
2. Resistance to insulin ↑
3. Glucose tolerance ↓

. . . .

Effects of ↑CHO Intake

1. Modify above responses
2. ↑Insulin/Glucagon
3. ↑Serum Triglycerides

increase in plasma insulin. There is also a resistance to insulin and a decrease in glucose tolerance (see Table 7-4). The mechanism of this resistance to insulin has not been completely solved to date. There are a number of studies (Salans, Knittle and Hirsch, 1967, 1968) suggesting that in most obese subjects there is an increase in the size of the adipocyte. There is a correlation between the sensitivity of the adipocyte and a decrease in size, so that as the adipocyte increases in size, it becomes less sensitive to insulin. If an obese person or a diabetic loses weight, there is a loss in the amount of lipid in the adipocyte. The adipocyte shrinks and at the same time the sensitivity to insulin increases. The effect of increasing the carbohydrate intake of the diet modifies this response but cannot completely account for it (Sims, Bray, Danforth, Glennon, Horton, Salans and O'Connell, 1974). That is, it is possible to demonstrate insulin resistance and a decreased glucose tolerance in the obese person even when on a low carbohydrate diet.

The peripheral resistance to insulin as adipocytes increase in size leads to a compensatory increase in insulin secretion, i.e., since the large adipocytes are less sensitive to insulin. In order to compensate for this decrease in sensitivity the pancreas produces more insulin, resulting in a higher level of circulating insulin. Insulin is known to increase lipogenesis or the synthesis of fatty acids in the liver. As fatty acid synthesis is increased, and as an excess of these substances are produced, they are diverted into the synthesis of more triglyceride, which then becomes available for the synthesis of VLDL. This sequence of events could lead to an increased synthesis of VLDL by the liver and to endogenous hypertriglyceridemia. The ratio of insulin to glucagon secretion depends, among other things, on the presence of obesity and the total calories and proportion of carbohydrates in the diet. When normal subjects are fed a high carbohydrate diet, the ratio of insulin to glucagon secretion increases, and there is a concomitant increase in the level of serum triglycerides and VLDL (Fujita, Gotto and Unger, 1975).

SUMMARY

In conclusion, there are at least six different types of primary hyperlipidemia phenotypes (World Health Organization, 1970) with different constellations of clinical manifestations and different responses to diet and obesity. The classification of the hyperlipidemias is based on which family of plasma lipoproteins is elevated. The triglyceride-rich families, the chylomicrons and VLDL, are particularly susceptible to obesity. Endogenous and exogenous hypertriglyceridemia are greatly exacerbated by obesity, probably due in part to an increased hepatic synthesis of VLDL. Hypercholesterolemia does not correspond well with degree of obesity. In obesity, the increased peripheral synthesis of cholesterol is not reflected in plasma hypercholesterolemia. Obesity directly and indirectly affects several of the risk factors for atherosclerosis including hyperlipidemia, hypertension, diabetes mellitus and physical activity.

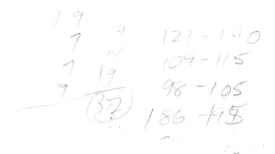

Chapter 8

Nutrition During Weight Loss

Lynne W. Scott, John P. Foreyt, and Antonio M. Gotto, Jr.

Obesity, in simplest terms, occurs because the caloric value of food ingested is greater than the body's energy expenditure. It has been said that no condition is easier to diagnose and more difficult to treat than obesity. In theory it seems simple, but in practice it may take years of hard conscientious work. There is no magic formula for weight reduction and the final outcome is the result of personal commitment and dietary adherence.

Dr. Charlotte Young (1960), a medical nutritionist at Cornell University, has studied successful dieters and has shown that those most likely to succeed have the following characteristics:

1. Personal motivation for weight loss or a reason to be thin.
2. Emotional stability.
3. Individual is not experiencing a time of stress.
4. Fat as an adult, but not as a child.
5. Ability to exert willpower to control fundamental human behavior, i.e., eating, drinking, and activity patterns.

The role of nutrition in weight reduction programs cannot be overemphasized. To work successfully with obese individuals, the therapist must be armed with a knowledge of the nutritive and

This work was supported by Grant No. HL 17269 from the National Heart and Lung Institute for the National Research and Demonstration Center.

caloric values of foods, as well as of energy needs and expenditures of individuals under various circumstances. It is also important to recognize the many nonmetabolic, nonnutritional uses of food, such as serving as rewards, replacement, or compensations for emotional stresses (Bruch, 1973). McReynolds' study (Chapter 4) substantiates the efficacy of using nutritionists trained in the principles and procedures of behavior modification as therapists in behavioral weight-loss programs. In programs of this nature the nutritionist works with individuals on techniques of *how* to reduce total caloric intake, in addition to the application of behavior modification techniques.

Diet used for weight reduction should follow the fundamental principles of nutrition. These fundamentals are very compatible with principles used to manage hyperlipidemia and obesity, two of the risk factors associated with heart disease, as discussed by Dr. Gotto in Chapter 7.

Guidelines for any diet aiming at control of hyperlipidemia or obesity should include:

1. Calories sufficient to permit physical vigor.
2. Protein sufficient for building and repairing body tissues and for growth.
3. Vitamins and minerals to regulate body processes.
4. Decreased saturated fat.
5. Increased polyunsaturated fat.
6. Reduced cholesterol intake.
7. Meets Recommended Dietary Allowances of essential nutrients.

The Recommended Dietary Allowances (RDA) of the Food and Nutrition Board, National Academy of Sciences-National Research Council, are standards used in the United States to provide guidance in planning diets. They are nutrient allowances, expressed as the daily nutrient intakes, judged to be necessary to maintain good nutrition in practically all healthy persons. The RDA are updated about every five years based on the research that has accumulated since the publication of the previous edition. The latest revision, in 1974, included zinc as a nutrient to be considered in planning diets (National Academy of Sciences, 1974).

In any diet, the best protection against nutritional inadequacy is a wide variety of food supplying the essential nutrients. One of the most rapidly growing areas of nutrition research is that of trace elements (Weininger and Briggs, 1974). Schwarz (1974) points out that "each newly discovered essential trace element opens up new prospects for biochemical and medical research."

For an individual to lose weight, an imbalance between caloric expenditure and caloric consumption must be achieved. Basal metabolism accounts for the largest quantity of energy expenditure and is usually related to body surface. Metabolic rate decreases as one grows older, and increases during pregnancy (as much as 20 percent over the basal rate prior to pregnancy). Studies have shown that starvation can result in a reduction of basal metabolic rate to less than 50 percent of prestarvation rate (Grande, Anderson, Taylor and Keys, 1957). The second largest component of caloric expenditure is energy related to activity. It is difficult to greatly increase total energy expenditure by activity, except for brief periods.

Weight Loss Diets

With perhaps 80,000,000 people in the United States being overweight or obese (Stuart and Davis, 1972), it is not surprising that discussions of calories and weight loss diets rank near the top of current topics for conversation. Although the scientific information on calories is known, it appears that the public has *not* been convinced that these facts hold the answer to the obesity problem. Diets for weight loss continue to appear with alleged scientific information for the public. Books advocating the "Easy Happy Effortless Way to Weight Loss" have been popular for years. Most of these diets ignore the basic fundamentals of nutrition and usually do not consider cholesterol and saturated fat in their diet plans. Young (1972) says that the most successful low-calorie diets fulfill the following criteria:

1. The diet should provide all of the nutrition which the body needs, except calories.

2. The diet should come as close as possible to the individual's normal habits of eating.

3. The diet should protect the individual from between-meal hunger, give a sense of well-being, and not cause a tired feeling.

4. The diet should enable the individual to eat at home and away from home without feeling as if everyone is staring at him.

5. The diet should be one that can be lived with for the rest of the individual's new thin life.

Popular "fad" diets range in scope from those which are totally carbohydrate to those containing very little carbohydrate. As far back as 1872, William Harvey published a diet for obesity that specifically indicted sweet and starchy foods, while permitting meat in *ad libitum* amounts. Variations of the low carbohydrate diet have reappeared periodically since that time. In 1953, Pennington wrote *Treatment of Obesity with Calorically Unrestricted Diets;* in 1960, the *Air Force Diet* (Air Force Diet, 1960) appeared; in 1961, Taller wrote *Calories Don't Count;* and in 1964, the *Drinking Man's Diet* (Jameson and Williams, 1964) became popular. More recent versions of the low carbohydrate diet include Stillman and Baker's (1967) *The Doctor's Quick Weight Loss Diet* and *Dr. Atkins' Diet Revolution: The High Calorie Way to Stay Thin Forever* (Atkins, 1972). Most of these diets focus on diet composition, placing special emphasis on carbohydrate restriction, but ignoring calorie content. Consequently, these diets are very high in protein and fat. One reason that these diets achieve any degree of weight loss at all is because individuals following them usually do not eat as many calories as previously consumed. A diet without carbohydrate, e.g., fruit, juice, vegetables, bread, and cereals, is rather boring.

Authors of the low carbohydrate diets promote the idea that diets low in carbohydrate generate sufficient ketone bodies ("incompletely burned" fat) to cause urinary losses of ketones in amounts large enough to account for weight losses in spite of high calorie intake. The amount of ketones lost in the urine rarely exceeds 100 kcal per day, a quantity that could not account for the dramatic results claimed for such diets.

Several potential hazards exist for individuals adhering to a diet very low in carbohydrate and rich in fat. According to the

American Medical Association's Council on Foods and Nutrition (1973), the greatest danger is related to hyperlipidemia, which may be induced by this regimen. Hyperlipidemia is one of the three major risk factors associated with heart disease. In one of the suggested menus in *Dr. Atkins' Diet Revolution* (1972), the cholesterol content is approximately 1850 mg, a level greater than four times that recommended, and it has a ratio of polyunsaturated fat to saturated fat of .1, which is below recommended standards (Inter-Society Commission for Heart Disease Resources, Atherosclerosis and Epidemiology Study Groups, 1970). Other hazardous effects caused by very low carbohydrate diets include increased levels of blood uric acid concentrations, fatigue, and low blood pressure (Bloom and Azar, 1963). *Dr. Atkin's Diet Revolution* (1972) states that the diet promotes the production of "fat mobilizing hormone" (FMH). According to Atkins, FMH releases energy into the bloodstream by causing the stored fat to convert to carbohydrates. No such hormone has been identified in man; fat is mobilized when insulin secretion diminishes (Cahill, 1971).

A *high* carbohydrate diet is the Zen Macrobiotic Diet (White, 1971). It is rooted in ancient Buddhist practices and divides foods into Yin and Yang. Accordingly, such foods as sugar and most fruits are Yin; meats, eggs, and such are Yang. The idea is to balance the menu by eating five Yins for every Yang. Brown rice has just about this ratio, which makes it the central element of the macrobiotic diet. It is potentially a very hazardous diet and the death of several individuals has been attributed to it.

A weight loss diet is considered "safe" only if it meets the Recommended Dietary Allowances (RDA). On an out-patient basis, it is very difficult to follow a diet below 1000 calories; such diets are often deficient in calcium or protein. Tullis (1973) says that emphasis should be placed on a daily caloric intake which permits a program of physical activity. This is generally at least a 1200-calorie diet.

The ideal ratio of carbohydrate, protein, and fat to total calories is 40-45 percent carbohydrate, 20 percent protein, and 35-40 percent fat. Werner (1955) showed that obese subjects on a low-carbohydrate diet, apart from transient changes in water balance, experience a weight loss similar to obese subjects on a "balanced" diet equal in caloric value.

Diets which recommend fasting and extremely low caloric levels are very difficult for patients to follow. Reports of follow-up results suggest that periods of fasting do not produce lasting weight loss superior to that obtained with conventional treatment (Innes, Campbell, Campbell, Needle, and Munro, 1974). Diets which recommend very low calorie levels usually revolve around counting calories. Keeping track of calories is a bothersome task for most individuals, one which is not usually continued over a long period of time. Examples of these diets include the *Computer Diet* (1965), and numerous others for which calories must be added up daily.

The food exchange method is more convenient to use than the calorie counting method. Five food exchange lists (Meat, Fruit, Bread, Dairy, and Fat) similar to those developed for diabetics (American Dietetic Association and American Diabetes Association, 1956) are usually used. Within each list various foods are specified and are approximately equal in calories to the other foods in that list. If one food is exchanged for another within the list, the calories are similar, thus making it possible to add variety to the weight reduction diet. A specified number of servings are allowed from each group daily (e.g., 6 Meat, 3 Fruit, 5 Bread, 2 Dairy, 8 Fat). Food exchanges are fairly easy to learn and can be applied without day-to-day calculations. The food exchange method allows a diet at a specific caloric level to be very quickly personalized to an individual's life style and nutritionally well-balanced.

Low Cholesterol Modified Fat Diet

The Prudent Heart Diet (Bennett and Simon, 1973) is a nutritionally well-balanced diet designed to manage two of the blood lipids—cholesterol and triglycerides. The calorie content can be modified to make it either a weight reduction or maintenance diet. This diet is called several different names. The American Heart Association (1972) calls it "The Way to a Man's Heart." For use in the Baylor College of Medicine National Heart and Blood Vessel Research and Demonstration Center, it is called the "HELP

Your Heart Eating Plan" (Gotto, Scott, Foreyt, and Reeves, 1975). All of these diets contain the same basic prescription. The Prudent Heart Diet is recommended by (1) The American Medical Association's Council on Foods and Nutrition, (2) the Food and Nutrition Board of the National Academy of Sciences National Research Council, and (3) the Intersociety Commission for Heart Disease Resources of the American Heart Association. The diet makes four recommendations to the general public:

1. Attain and maintain desirable body weight.
2. Decrease intake of saturated fat.
3. Increase intake of polyunsaturated fat.
4. Lower cholesterol consumption.

It consists of 300 to 500 mg of cholesterol and has a polyunsaturated fat to saturated fat ratio (P/S) of 1.0. (The average American consumes from 200 mg to 2000 mg of cholesterol daily and his diet has an average P/S ratio of about 0.3.)

Wilson, Hulley, Burrows, and Nichaman (1971) demonstrated that the Prudent Heart Diet can lower serum cholesterol by 10 percent, triglycerides by 12 percent, and the other lipoproteins including pre-beta-lipoprotein by 6 percent and beta-lipoprotein by 16 percent. This diet is nutritionally adequate and easy for people to follow on an out-patient basis over an extended period of time. The "Anti-Coronary Club" (Christakis et al., 1966) demonstrated that individuals following the Prudent Heart Diet effectively lowered serum cholesterol within the first year and maintained the lowered levels up to six years, at which time the study ended. The average serum cholesterol fell from 260 mg/100 ml to 228 mg/100 ml and remained at that level. The Framingham study (Cornfield, 1970) suggests that a 10 percent reduction in the serum cholesterol levels of the population would yield a 23 percent decrease in the incidence of heart disease.

The first objective of the Prudent Heart Diet, weight control, is very compatible with the other three, decreased intake of saturated fat, increased intake of polyunsaturated fat, and reduced cholesterol consumption. Research studies show that saturated fat tends to increase levels of serum cholesterol; polyunsaturated fat tends to decrease serum cholesterol; and monounsaturated fat has

TABLE 8-1

Ratio of Polyunsaturated to
Saturated Fats

Safflower	9.0
Corn	5.3
Sunflower	5.3
Soybean	3.5
Cottonseed	2.0
Peanut	1.6
Olive	.63
Lard	.3
Palm	.2
Butter	.1
Coconut	.02

Adapted from *Fatty Acids in Food Fats*, Home
Eco. Research Report #7, U.S.D.A., 1959, and
from *Fats and Oils, Fatty Acid Composition and
Physical Properties*, Drew Chemical Corporation,
Parsippany, N. J.

no effect on the level of serum cholesterol. Keys, Anderson, and
Grande (1965) showed that the addition of 2 gm polyunsaturated
fat to the diet is approximately equivalent in cholesterol-lowering
effect to the removal of 1 gm of saturated fat. In a 12-year study
recently reported in Finland, Miettinen, Turpeinen, Karvonen,
and Elosuo (1972) reported that an average reduction of serum
cholesterol of 12 to 18 percent was achieved by two relatively
simple dietary modifications: 1) butter was replaced by a "soft"
margarine with a high P/S ratio, and 2) the substitution of "filled"
milk for whole milk. The "filled" milk was an emulsion of soybean
oil in skim milk.

Dietary Fat

Since fat plays such an important role in the control of serum
cholesterol and weight, it is important to understand how the fats
differ. The ratio of polyunsaturated fat to saturated fat (P/S
ratio) is determined by dividing the polyunsaturated fatty acids
by the saturated fatty acids. Monounsaturated fatty acids are not
included. The higher the P/S ratio, the better the fat. Table 8-1
shows the P/S ratio for the most commonly used fats. Safflower
oil has a P/S of 9, followed by corn and sunflower oil. Peanut oil

and olive oil are examples of monounsaturated fat. Palm, coconut, lard, and butter are forms of saturated fat. For similar amounts of the different fats, i.e., oil, margarine, butter, and lard, each has similar calories. Since the P/S ratios of fats vary, those having the highest P/S ratio should constitute the largest percentage of fat in the diet.

Saturated fats are usually solid at room temperature and are usually of animal origin. Examples of saturated fats include butter, lard, meat fat, the butterfat in dairy products, and solid shortenings. Two fats from plant origin, coconut and palm kernel oil, are saturated fats. These short-chain fatty acids are very stable and have a long shelf life. They do not break down and become rancid when combined with other foods. Coconut and palm kernel oil are used quite extensively in non-dairy products, such as coffee creamers, whipped toppings, and sour cream substitutes.

Polyunsaturated fats are of plant origin and are liquid at room temperature. These fats are highest in polyunsaturated fatty acids in the liquid state.

Margarines can be a good source of polyunsaturated fat if liquid safflower, corn, or sunflower oil is the first ingredient listed on the label. Tub margarines have a higher percentage of oil than stick margarines and therefore usually have a higher P/S ratio. "Diet" margarines list water as the first ingredient. The second ingredient in order of predominance is usually "hydrogenated" or "partially hardened" fat. The term "hydrogenation" means that hydrogen atoms have been added to the molecule thus making it more of a saturated fat. The preferable first ingredient should be a "liquid" fat.

Monounsaturated fats do not affect the level of serum cholesterol, but have the same caloric value for equivalent amounts of saturated and polyunsaturated fats. Examples of monounsaturated fats are olives, olive oil, peanut butter, peanut oil, avocados, and most nuts. These fats are allowed on cholesterol controlled diets.

Dietary Cholesterol

The recommended level of cholesterol is 300 to 500 mg per day. In our society, the daily ingestion of cholesterol may be much higher, varying from 200 to 2000 mg per day. Cholesterol is

TABLE 8-2
Cholesterol Content

Food	Amount	Mg. Chol.
Egg yolk	1	252
Liver (chicken)	3 oz	636
Liver (beef, hog, lamb)	3 oz	372
Shrimp	3 oz (6 large or 15 small)	128
Veal, lean	3 oz	86
Cheese, Cheddar	3 oz	84
Beef, lean	3 oz	77
Pork, lean	3 oz	76
Chicken, breast (without skin)	3 oz	68
Fish (flounder, halibut, haddock, cod) raw	3 oz	48
Milk—whole	1 cup	34
low fat	1 cup	22
skim	1 cup	5
Fruits and vegetables		0

Adapted from Feeley, R. M., Criner, P. E., Watt, B. K., Cholesterol Content of Foods. *Journal of the American Dietetic Association,* 1972, 61, 134.

present in the diet of all individuals who eat or drink foods of animal origin. For practical purposes, we do not consider plants to have cholesterol; however, trace amounts have been reported in a few samples of plant tissues. The peak of cholesterol absorption takes place 6 to 9 hours after eating. The absorption of cholesterol is not complete. Only about 50 percent of that ingested is actually absorbed. The absorption of cholesterol depends on the size of the dose; with increasing amounts eaten, the percentage absorbed decreases, although the actual amount increases. The quantity of cholesterol, as well as the P/S ratio of the diet, exerts a significant influence on serum cholesterol.

Foods highest in cholesterol include egg yolk, liver, and crayfish. Table 8-2 shows the cholesterol value of some common foods. There has been a strong tendency, although not completely correct, to consider cholesterol content in food to be related to the fat content and to assume that by removing fat, cholesterol would be proportionately reduced. Calories and saturated fat are reduced by the removal of fat, but cholesterol remains unaffected.

FIGURE 8-1

SATURATED FAT AND POLYUNSATURATED FAT IN BEEF, POULTRY, AND FISH

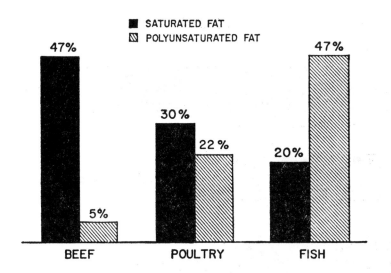

Figure 8-1 shows a comparison between saturated fat and polyunsaturated fat in beef, poultry, and fish. Beef contains a high percentage of saturated fats (47 percent) and a very low percentage of polyunsaturated fats (5 percent). Poultry is somewhat lower in saturated fat (30 percent) and is much higher in polyunsaturated fat than beef. Fish has only 20 percent saturated fat and 47 percent polyunsaturated fat, or more than twice as much polyunsaturated fat as saturated fat. Figure 8-2 shows how the calories vary for beef, poultry, and fish. Fish has about half the calories of beef. It is also naturally lower in fat than beef.

The HELP Your Heart Eating Plan (Gotto, Scott, Foreyt, and Reeves, 1975) takes the fundamentals of good nutrition, the kind of fat, cholesterol, and calories into consideration and recommends the following:

1. Meat, fish, or poultry—7 ounces daily.
2. Egg yolks—2 weekly.

Figure 8-2

CALORIES IN BEEF, POULTRY, AND FISH

4 OZ. SERVING

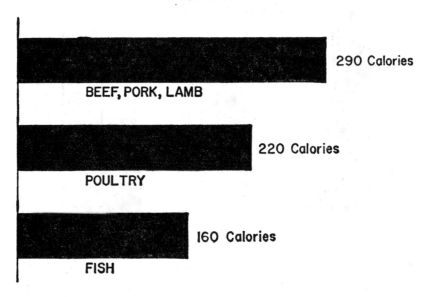

290 Calories

BEEF, PORK, LAMB

220 Calories

POULTRY

160 Calories

FISH

3. Polyunsaturated oil—2 tablespoons daily.
4. Soft safflower or corn oil margarine—2 tablespoons daily.
5. Dairy products—2 servings daily.
6. Bread and cereals—4 or more servings daily.
7. Fruits and vegetables—4 or more servings daily.

In selecting meat, the leanest cuts, with a minimum of marbling (i.e., the fat dispersed through the lean tissue), are recommended. All visible fat should be trimmed before cooking. Most preparation methods are acceptable—roasting, broiling, charcoaling, grilling, braising, stewing, and even frying, if the calories are taken into consideration and a polyunsaturated oil is used.

The HELP Your Heart Eating Plan recommends two egg yolks

Table 8-3

Alcohol

Any one of the following is a serving:

1   ounce gin, rum, vodka or whiskey
1½   ounces dessert or sweet wine
2½   ounces dry table wine
5   ounces beer

a week including those used in cooking. Egg substitutes without cholesterol can be used if additional "eggs" are desired.

Although the HELP Your Heart Eating Plan recommends two tablespoons each of polyunsaturated oil and margarine, the amount is reduced if weight is a problem.

The dairy products are the best sources of calcium and phosphorus, essential nutrients for strong, healthy bones and teeth. Dairy products are also a source of high quality protein. Since dairy products are a source of saturated fat, only the fat-free and low-fat products are recommended. Two cups of low-fat (2 percent butterfat) milk are allowed; however, for even greater cholesterol-lowering effect, skim milk is recommended. As an exchange for milk, cheeses made from skim milk or those with less than 8 percent butterfat can be used in the diet. Nutritionally this is a very important food group and one which many low calorie diets neglect to emphasize.

The bread and cereal products provide some of the essential vitamins and minerals. Selections should be from either those which are whole grain or "enriched." The food exchange list method classifies the starchy vegetables (potatoes, corn, etc.), the pastas (spaghetti, macaroni, etc.), simple desserts (angel food cake, sherbet, plain puddings) and alcohol (no more than two servings per day, see Table 8-3) into the bread and cereal group. Although not all of these foods are grain products, it is possible to exchange the calories in specified amounts.

Fruits and vegetables contain many essential vitamins and minerals needed by the body. For calorie control diets, unsweetened fruits should be used. An exchange list allows a wide variety of fruits and juices to be included in specified amount. Green vegetables, such as broccoli, green beans, asparagus, and salad greens

Table 8-4
Tips for Eating Out

CHOOSE FROM THESE ITEMS

First Course: Clear soup
Tomato juice
Fresh fruit cup

Main Course: Fish, chicken, beef
(baked or broiled without additional fat)
Sliced turkey or veal
London broil (flank steak) without gravy
Fish salad
Cottage cheese/fruit plate

Vegetables: Tossed salad with oil and vinegar dressing or French
dressing
Baked potato with margarine, chives, imitation bacon
Cooked or raw vegetables without butter

Dessert: Fresh fruit
Sherbet
Gelatin
Angel food cake without frosting

SAY "NO" TO THESE ITEMS

First Course: Cream soups

Main Course: Fried meat
Casseroles
Creamed foods

Vegetables: Fried vegetables
Cheese sauces

Desserts: Pie
Ice cream
Cake
Pudding

Miscellaneous: Butter
Cheese dressing
Sour cream
Bacon

are low in calories and are good to "fill up" on for individuals needing to lose weight. These can be eaten either raw or cooked. Weight reduction programs such as The Mouthful Diet (Fowler, Fordyce, Boyd, and Masock, 1972) which require that chews be counted daily and strive for increasingly fewer chews fail to recognize that some of the foods needing the most chewing such as celery, carrots, and other raw vegetables are the lowest in calories.

The HELP Your Heart Eating Plan can be used for either a weight reduction diet or a maintenance diet. Maintenance is the "key" to any weight reduction diet; there is no advantage to losing weight if it is regained. All diets, whether for weight reduction or maintenance, should present an eating plan that is flexible enough to accommodate individual life style. Table 8-4 is a list of suggestions for those who eat out.

Conclusion

The principles of nutrition, as well as those associated with diet and heart disease, low cholesterol, and modified fat, should always be taken into consideration in weight loss programs. These basic principles of diet are very compatible with those taught by behavioral psychologists and should never be neglected in weight reduction programs.

Chapter 9

Training Nutrition Educators: Behavior Modification in the Kitchen

Valerie B. Knotts

"Welcome to Behavior Modification! You are going to be involved in an exciting experiment in nutrition education; an attempt to give you individualized instruction within the confines of a regular class." This was the introduction to a self-paced course in Behavior Modification offered to graduate students in nutrition.

The use of behavior modification in the treatment of obesity has gained much attention recently, as a novel way to treat one of the nation's major health problems. The TODAY television show featured a week-long series in which the problem and treatment of obesity was presented. Among the various methods discussed, behavior modification seemed to hold the most promise as a way of bringing overweight under control and maintaining weight loss over a period of time.

Since overweight is directly related to what an individual eats each day, the general practice has been to recommend a weight reduction diet as a means of treatment. However, the success rate using diet alone has been rather dismal. Many people have tried this method only to regain what was lost and in some cases to gain back more weight than before they went on the diet. Over years of following this practice, one may gain and lose the same twenty-five to fifty pounds several times, thus displaying what is known as the "yo-yo effect," which can be a serious hazard to health.

A distinct characteristic of behavior modification is the belief that behavior disorders are learned responses and that modern learning theories have much to teach us regarding both the acquisition and extinction of these responses (Eysenck, 1963). At Lifestyle, a weight reduction center in Los Angeles, Marston and London have studied the eating habits of both overweight and thin people. The critical factor seems to be the way people eat, more so than what they eat. Thin people chew their food longer and more slowly, and often leave food on their plate. Fat people eat more, drink more, eat faster, chew faster and even less, clean their plate, and probably enjoy food less. Marston and London are convinced that overweight people can be trained to eat like thin people. It takes commitment, hard work, self-assessment, and systematic record keeping to change eating habits. Though an overweight person may never become like a thin person, he can develop a new set of habits which can give him self-control over his eating problem.

One of the first considerations in a behavior modification program is behavioral analysis. It begins with a study of the environmental variables which control an individual's eating behavior. These events or variables can be separated into antecedent events, those which occur before eating, and consequent events, those which serve to maintain or reward eating behavior. Ferster, Nurnberger, and Levitt (1962) recommended the restructuring of the eating environment. Stuart (1971) summarized these recommendations and has used them as the basis for much of his work in treating obesity.

The environment most often needing to be changed is that in which the individual consumes food. Subjects were asked to record what they ate, where, with whom, and how they felt at the time. From this diary it was learned that overweight people ate while watching television, while reading, while in the kitchen cooking, because they were bored, and often as a reward. As a part of treatment, subjects have been asked to eat in the same place, using a smaller plate, to chew the food longer and slower, and to place the knife and fork on the plate between bites instead of holding them. Eating should be a pure experience, without additional distractions of reading or watching television, if eating habits are to be reprogrammed.

Studies based on the reprogramming of the environment have shown the best results of any of the behavior modification approaches. Most subjects regularly lost small amounts of weight during treatment and maintained the weight loss after treatment ended (Stuart, 1973).

Based on the belief that behavior modification can be a very effective educational technique, plans were made to include a course in behavior modification in the education component of the graduate program in nutrition. Treatment of obesity is probably one of the most common reasons why people are referred to a dietitian for counseling and weight reduction. Since results obtained from diet alone have been rather discouraging, the need for a new approach was obvious. Use of behavior modification offers an approach with demonstrated positive results supported by a number of research studies.

Fifteen students enrolled for the first offering of the course in behavior modification. The development of the course outline and the use of a self-paced format was the outgrowth of a course which the instructor had taken previously at another university. The ideas and method of presentation were adapted from those used by Dr. Sander Martin (1973).

The course was divided into four sections. The first two sections covered the terminology and procedures used in behavior modification, and the text chosen was *Behavior Principles* (Ferster and Perrott, 1968). In the introduction, the authors devoted considerable space to the concept of mastery learning and how it was applied in using the book. The method is based on the work of F. S. Keller (1967) and others who worked with students to develop the technique of mastering one part before continuing on to the next. The concepts of presentation are related to those of programmed teaching, but as the authors suggest, they have extended them to a much broader application.

The key to mastery learning is in the interview technique, in which the student must interact with peers and with the instructor in discussing the probe questions. The student fulfills the role of the interviewee first in explaining the material; when this has been evaluated as complete and satisfactory, he switches roles and becomes the interviewer. As the interviewer, he must serve as a skilled listener in evaluating the interviewee's behavior and providing encouragement. Advancement to the next unit is contingent upon the student's ability to discuss the material in a knowledgeable manner indicating that he understands its meaning and importance. In essence, the interview serves as a reinforcer which shapes and maintains the study behavior that leads to mastery of the subject and the acquisition of the technical vocabulary.

When participating in the interview, the student is allowed to use the text. The primary concern is not how well he has memorized the material, but how well he can paraphrase, or discuss in his own words, the meaning of the material. From experience, those students who demonstrated the most skill in discussing the material in their own words had the least difficulty in responding to the questions on the written tests at the end of each section. A common remark made by the students indicated that they really did not need to study the questions before writing the test, since they had covered them so well in the interview sessions.

The class was small, so no student assistants were available, as suggested by Keller (1967). However, an adaptation of this procedure was achieved by having the instructor serve as the interviewer for about one-third of the class. These students then acted as interviewers. Each student was required to have a successful interview on a chapter before he could interview another student on the same material. So that students were not interviewing the same people each time, they were limited in the number of interviews they could conduct with the same person, except the instructor. If, at the end of a unit, some students still needed to listen to an interview, but all had been interviewed, then two students were paired and asked to respond to alternating questions.

For the third section, another text was chosen, *Control of Human Behavior: From Cure to Prevention, Vol. 2* (Ulrich, Stachnik, and Mabry, 1970). Having learned the terminology and techniques in the first two sections, the emphasis was shifted to the application of behavior modification techniques in a variety of situations. The authors described the successful development of behavioral technology from both the experimental and applied analysis of behavior. The volume was intended to be compatible with basic texts on behavior modification and served as a valuable extension to *Behavior Principles*.

Students were introduced to the scientific analysis of behavior, remediation of behavioral problems in institutional and non-institutional settings, and prevention of future behavior problems. Of particular significance was the collection of articles which discussed the issues and implications of using operant conditioning and the ethical considerations involved. For students learning to use behavior modification, it is essential to be aware of the ethical and legal implications, and to assume responsibility for the appropriate, wise, and humane use of such techniques.

Two color films were used to supplement the reading materials for the course. The first film was presented after the third week, which allowed the students the opportunity to acquire some of the basic concepts of behavior modification and learning theory. The film *Learning* (produced by Carol Hart for CRM, 1961) demonstrated how people learn by showing examples of the classical conditioning model used by Watson and Rayner in conditioning a child to fear white furry objects, the operant-reinforcement model applying contingency management, and the principles of generalization. Psychologist B. F. Skinner also discussed his model of operant conditioning. The timing for presenting the first film was important, because at about the fourth week students are somewhat overwhelmed by the terminology and experimental orientation of the material. The film provided the opportunity to see some of the techniques applied to animals and humans, and reinforced the importance of understanding the procedures and vocabulary.

During section three the second film was shown, *One Step at a Time: An Introduction to Behavior Modification* (produced by Roger Ulrich for CRM, 1973). This film was an important extension of the work in *Control of Human Behavior*. Positive reinforcement using praise, physical contact, tokens, charts and graphs, and other rewards was demonstrated with handicapped children, children with learning problems, and disturbed adults. Other films are available, but these seemed the most appropriate for enhancing the mastery learning approach of the course.

After completion of each of the first three sections, students were asked to write an exam consisting of ten to twelve questions randomly selected from the probe questions used for the interview sessions. A score of 80 percent was required, and students were asked to repeat the written exam if they failed to meet the 80 percent criterion. A different set of questions were selected when repeat exams were necessary. For this class, only one student had to repeat a test and that was the first written exam. For the remaining tests, all students scored 80 percent or above on the first attempt.

The fourth section of the course was labeled as the application portion. *Slim Chance in a Fat World* (Stuart and Davis, 1972), was used as an example of a successful behavioral control program. Students had two options from which to choose. They could develop a behavioral control program and implement it where feasible, or they could research some aspect of behavioral therapy from the current literature and present it as a seminar. A sampling of the projects included several reports on behavior therapy programs for obesity and for anorexia nervosa, an investigation of the ethical issues in using behavior modification, and a report of a visit to observe in a private day school serving children with learning disabilities, where contingency management was used.

Two projects which grew out of the application section of the course deserve further comment. Two students* working as dietitians for a private medical clinic developed a Weight Management Program to be used with individual patients. Several factors were considered in designing the program:

1. The clinic has a large private group practice of physicians located in one building with complete diagnostic facilities available.
2. Obese patients, seen by the clinic dietitians, are referred by the patient's physician because obesity is a contributing factor in the patient's medical problem.
3. Most of the obese patients have tried a variety of diets with little or no success and have been unable to maintain their desired weight.
4. Most of the patients seen at the clinic are able to afford,

---

* The dietitians who have developed the weight management program are Ms. Tyra Kane and Ms. Barbara Norman, both graduate students in the College of Nutrition, Texas Woman's University, Houston, Texas.

TABLE 9-1

Age, Marital Status, Weight Loss, Time, and
Number of Sessions for Six Male Patients

Patient	Age	Marital Status	Initial Weight (lbs.)	Weight Loss to Date	Time (weeks)	Sessions to Date
1	24	S	199	—24	17	3
2	34	M	234	— 7	8	2
3	51	S	219	—17	8	2
4	49	S	248	— 6	4	3
5	44	M	240	—55*	26	5
6	52	M	305	—53	29	2

* Patient reached weight loss goal.

and are willing to pay for, any services they need or
desire.

5. Because of the patient's income and social involvement,
many are not willing to join a group type management
program where they publicly admit to their weight problem before people they do not know.

6. The typical clinic patient is accustomed to individual attention and recognition from many sources, and he expects
this same individualized, personal concern from the physician, the dietitian, and any other member of the health
care team involved in his treatment.

Initially, the Weight Management Program was tried on two
patients with the physician's consent, to see what kind of progress
could be achieved. One patient moved out of the city two months
later and no follow-up was possible. The other patient, a male
who weighed 240 pounds at the beginning of the treatment,
followed the program for a period of six months, during which
he lost a total of 55 pounds. At a follow-up period five months
after termination of treatment, he was maintaining his present
weight of 185. From the results achieved with this patient, the
dietitians were ready to present the Weight Management Program to the entire medical staff. The program has been in operation for approximately 10 months, including the initial portion.
Fifty patients have agreed to the terms of the program, and most
of these patients have been successful in losing weight and main-

FIGURE 9-1
Weight Profile for Patients 1-4 (Males) in
Weight Management Program

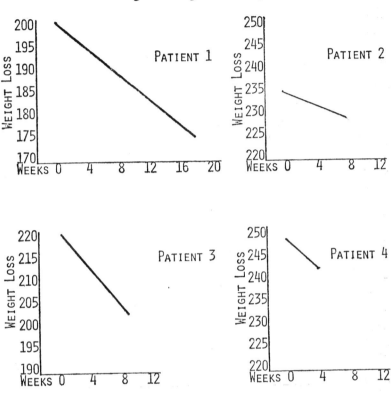

taining the weight loss. The success rate has been 100 percent with the male patients, but somewhat lower with the housewives and the teenagers, which is consistent with the literature.

Table 9-1 presents the age, marital status, initial weight, weight loss, time, and number of sessions for six males who participated in the weight management program. All were successful in losing weight. The weight loss ranged from —6 to —55 pounds with an average weight loss of —24.1 pounds. One patient reached his goal by the 26th week, and after 48 weeks is continuing to main-

FIGURE 9-2
Weight Profile for Patient 5 (Male) in
Weight Management Program

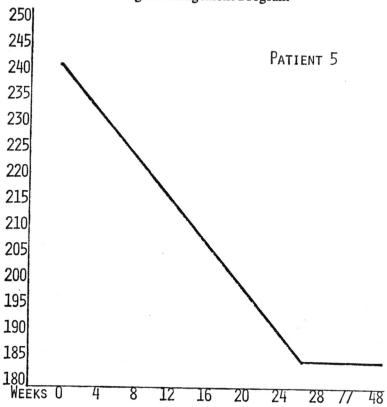

PATIENT 5

tain his weight loss (patient 5, Figure 9-2). The weight loss for each of the subjects is shown graphically in Figures 9-1, 9-2, and 9-3.

Figure 9-4 presents the weight profile for 22 females, ranging in age from 20-58 years, who participated in the weight management program. Because of the number of patients involved, the data are presented as the average weight loss to date, —6.3 pounds. The average number of visits is 2.8, and the length of time in the program ranges from 2 to 6 months.

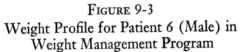

FIGURE 9-3
Weight Profile for Patient 6 (Male) in
Weight Management Program

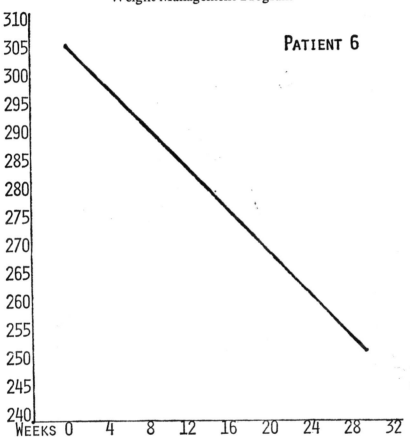

Table 9-2 presents the age, initial weight, weight loss, time, and number of sessions for each of four teenage female patients. The average weight loss was —6.6 pounds over an average of 3.25 sessions. In Figure 9-5, the weight profile for each of the teenagers is graphically displayed.

The response to the program by the physicians, in referring patients, and by the participants, in suggesting it to their friends,

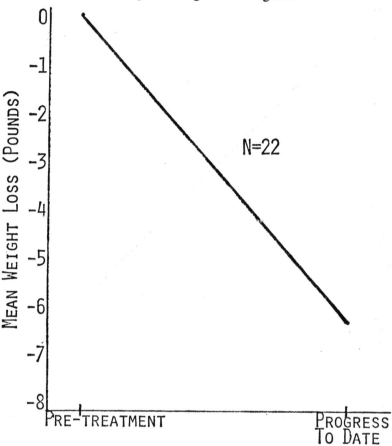

FIGURE 9-4
Weight Profile for Twenty-two Women Participating in
Weight Management Program

has been somewhat overwhelming. It has not allowed time to develop a system for easy retrieval of information, nor for statistical analysis of the results. This is now being done manually, but plans are underway to have computer access to the information very soon.

A second project worthy of comment was an experimental study in the treatment of obesity using behavior modification as

TABLE 9-2

Age, Weight Loss, Time, and Number of Sessions for Teenage Female Patients

Patient	Age	Initial Weight (lbs.)	Weight Loss to Date	Time in	Sessions to Date
1	15	200	— 3	21	3
2	14	152½	—11.5	8	2
3	17	170	—16	21	4
4	16	160	+ 4	17	4

FIGURE 9-5

Weight Profile for Four Teenage Females in Weight Management Program

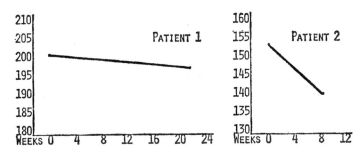

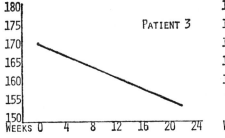

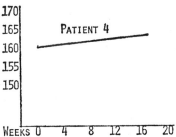

a teaching method. College students at a local university volunteered to participate in the study. Two groups were selected: one group met monthly for a weigh-in and discussion of a weight reduction diet (traditional method), and the second group met weekly for weigh-in and the behavior modification program. This program was conducted jointly by a nutritionist* and a psychologist from the university. Ten dollars was collected from each participant in the behavior modification group. This money was then divided into differing percentages and used to reinforce weight loss, following the diet, and record keeping. The percentages were larger after a special holiday (Thanksgiving), when weight loss would be more difficult. As part of the contract, the subjects agreed that any money not returned by the end of the program (seven weeks) would be donated to a scholarship fund. When the results of the two groups were compared, the subjects in the behavior modification program were found to have lost more weight than those following the traditional program, although the differences were not statistically significant.

Based on the favorable response from the students who enrolled in the behavior modification course, the decision was made to include it as a regular offering for the graduate program in nutrition. Students in the graduate nursing program have also indicated interest in learning more about behavior modification as a teaching method.

Generally, the response to the course format was favorable. However, some students who preferred the lecture method were not comfortable with the individualized interview approach. Their frustrations increased when they had to wait to complete an interview if the instructor or another student was not available when they wanted to be interviewed. This could be remedied by using graduate teaching assistants. Some expressed concern that there was too much theory and not enough practical application in the course. Since the course was offered at a graduate level, the theoretical foundation was considered essential to the understanding and wise application of the method. The real limitation was the time required to master the concepts of behavior modifica-

---

* Ms. Margaret Lovell is the nutritionist who developed this study; she is a graduate student in the College of Nutrition, Texas Woman's University, Houston, Texas.

tion. By the time mastery was accomplished, only three or four weeks remained to apply the technique to a practical situation. This did not allow sufficient time within the semester to complete the implementation and evaluation of a program.

All things considered, the inclusion of behavior modification in nutrition education has been a worthwhile endeavor. It offers real promise as a technique for the dietitian to use in helping people to achieve self-control over their eating habits.

Part IV

COMPREHENSIVE BEHAVIORAL TREATMENT PROGRAMS

INTRODUCTION

In Part IV, the diet modification programs at Stanford University Medical School, Duke University Medical School, and Baylor College of Medicine are presented and samples of their programs illustrated. Dr. James M. Ferguson, in Chapter 10, "A clinical program for the behavioral control of obesity," describes the Eating Disorders Clinic at Stanford, established by Dr. Albert Stunkard, following his pioneering work at the University of Pennsylvania. The program involves 40 weeks of treatment (two 20-week therapy periods) in group settings and can be administered by trained non-professionals. Ferguson presents data showing the efficacy of the program and discusses the problems and limitations involved in clinics like this one. The program is a good example of one using a total behavioral package, making use of all facets of the A B C paradigm discussed in earlier chapters.

The staff of the Stanford Eating Disorders Clinic present their questionnaire in Chapter 11, "A clinical and research questionnaire for obese patients." It should be of interest to those who have in operation plans to develop similar type programs.

In Chapter 12, "Affective and cognitive behavior change: Essential components of comprehensive obesity treatment," Dr. Gerard J. Musante describes the multimodal Dietary Rehabilitation Clinic at Duke University. Distinctive to this program is the large number of clients who have gross obesity and the extent to which these clients have been refractory to other treatment programs. Musante describes clearly the theoretical underpinnings of his program, along with the basic treatment program. He plans a major emphasis on the affective and *cognitive* aspects involved in weight control. Assertive training also plays an integral part in the treatment program.

In the final chapter, "Diet modification in the community," Dr. John P. Foreyt, Lynne W. Scott, and Dr. Antonio M. Gotto, Jr. emphasize not only the importance of weight control but also the control of serum lipids (cholesterol and triglycerides) because of their role as a risk factor in the development of cardiovascular diseases. The authors review the behavioral techniques used in weight control and point out many of the methodological problems involved. The Diet Modification Clinic directs itself to reduction of serum lipids and weight with the general public. Their HELP Your Heart Eating Plan, combined with behavioral techniques, is now being tested on large numbers of individuals to see whether the techniques are applicable and feasible for use with individuals who have "normal" lipids and who are not overweight (the idea being that "normal" lipids are too high in a society where heart disease is the number one killer).

These three programs provide the reader with examples of large ongoing programs where behavioral principles and techniques have been integrated into comprehensive treatment programs.

Chapter 10

A Clinical Program for the Behavioral Control of Obesity

James M. Ferguson

Obesity is a prevalent disorder of major concern to physicians in this country. Excess weight is associated with increased incidence, morbidity, and mortality from most major diseases (Thorn, 1970). Treatments for obesity have traditionally been very ineffective. Stunkard's pronouncement in 1959, "Most obese persons will not enter treatment, of those who do enter treatment, most will not lose weight, (and) of those who do lose weight, most will regain it" (Stunkard and McLaren-Hume, 1959), was quite accurate. Amphetamines, human chorionic gonadotropin with a 500-calorie diet, diguanides, thyroid analogs, hypnosis, diets, starvation, and exhortation all lead to weight loss in some patients. However, almost always this loss is followed by an equal or greater weight gain (Penick and Stunkard, 1972).

Several avenues of investigation have led to our current clinical program for weight control. One of the landmark experiments in the treatment of obesity was carried out in 1965 by London and

This research was supported in part by NIMH Grant MH 25568-01 awarded to Dr. A. J. Stunkard for the Clinical and Experimental Study of Human Obesity.

I would like to acknowledge the assistance of the staff of the Stanford Eating Disorders Clinic in this project: Drs. Albert Stunkard and W. Stewart Agras have provided faculty supervision for the Clinic, Drs. Joellen Werne, C. Barr Taylor, Charles Greaves, and Brandon Qualls have served as group leaders, and Ms. Janet Ruby, Ms. Carolyn Wright, and Dr. Colleen S. W. Rand have provided editorial comment throughout.

Schreiber (1966). When they studied the effects of drug and placebo medication in supportive groups and supportive individual treatment situations, they found a lower dropout rate and a greater weight loss for patients included in therapy groups regardless of drug or placebo medication treatment. This report was especially interesting because of the reported failure to obtain reliable weight loss in the context of the standard doctor-patient or psychotherapist-client relationship.

About the same time, Ferster suggested a learning approach to weight control (Ferster, Nurnberger and Levitt, 1962). His basic postulate was the existence of a difference in eating behaviors between obese and thin individuals. To combat this difference, he developed a behavior modification program to change overweight subjects' eating behaviors toward "normal." Stuart developed a treatment program based on Ferster's work, and published results in 1967 of a program for weight control which was more effective than any previously published outpatient treatment for obesity. He treated ten women individually for one year. Two patients dropped out of treatment. All of the remaining lost over 25 pounds, and four of the initial ten patients lost over 40 pounds. This was a small, highly selected, but dramatically successful group of patients.

The most systematic studies of the variables involved in weight loss and maintenance have been from Stunkard's group at the University of Pennsylvania (Stunkard, 1972; Westlake, Levitz and Stunkard, 1974; Stunkard and Mahoney, 1975). They combined group therapy with a behavioral approach and reported very significant weight losses. Over 50 percent of their patients lost more than 20 pounds, and 80 percent of these patients either maintained their lower weight or lost more weight during the subsequent two years.

During the past year, the Stanford Eating Disorders Clinic has developed a behavioral program for weight control which incorporates many of the elements of the Pennsylvania work along with subsequent developments reported in the scientific literature. Our goal has been to develop a systematic program that can be administered to groups of patients by relatively untrained individuals. A package of 20 weekly lessons has been written for use in this program. These lessons are taught to our patients in two

20-week therapy periods which are paid for separately. The therapy format is currently five weeks of instruction alternating with five weeks of maintenance or practice.

The lessons are:

1. Introduction to the behavioral control of weight: An overview of the principles of behavior modification and the first ten weeks of instruction.
2. Cue elimination: Exercises in stimulus narrowing, e.g., eating in one place, eliminating other activities while eating, removing food cues from the environment, etc.
3. Changing the act of eating: Slowing down the act of eating by putting eating utensils on the table between bites.
4. Behavioral chains and alternate activities: Substitution of alternate activities for antecedent behaviors.
5. Behavioral analysis, feedback, and maintenance: An introduction to problem solving.

M1 to M5: Five weeks of maintenance or practice, with optional weekly weighings at the Clinic.

6. Preplanning: Thinking ahead about meal content to take impulse out of eating.
7. Cue elimination part two, and Energy use part one: Stimulus narrowing associated with food, e.g., leaving food behind, throwing away leftovers, taking serving dishes off the table, etc. An activity baseline is obtained for one week with a pedometer.
8. Energy use part two: Systematic increase of energy expenditure.
9. Snacks, cues, and holidays: Hints for dealing with snacks and social situations, and a discussion of the caloric content of snacks.
10. Environmental support—family and friends: A discussion of family interactions and the need for support at home. Families are requested to attend this meeting.

M6 to M10: Five weeks of maintenance or practice, with optional weekly weighings at the clinic.

11. Progress, maintenance, feedback, and review: A session designed to provide feedback about maintenance, and review the first ten weeks.
12. The behavioral diet: An introduction to the Stuart and Davis (1972) food exchange diet.

13. Self Instruction I—becoming aware of internal dialogue: A baseline week of exercises to increase the awareness of cognitive processes.

14. Self instruction II—rescripting and reward: Instruction on how to change internal dialogue, and the principles of and need for self-reward.

15. Self instruction III—rescripting, reward, self-image, and maintenance: Self-image is presented as a key to maintenance, the need for systematic change of this image is stressed, and the use of self-reward to help make this change is introduced.

M11 to M15: Five weeks of maintenance or practice with optional weekly weighings at the Clinic.

16. Review, reattribution, and negative self-instruction: Introduction to positive attribution to hunger, negative attribution to satiety, and covert sensitization for problem foods.

17. Contingency contracting—making a deal with yourself: Contingency contracting on a day to day basis with practice specifying goals and rewards.

18. Contingency contracting with others: Long-term goals and rewards, and social involvement.

19. Social cues to eating—how to avoid them: Attribution of hunger to external cues, and dealing with social situations more directly with non-food related behaviors.

20. Final review, and discussion of maintenance.

Patient Selection

Our patients are both self-referred and physician-referred for weight reduction. As a prerequisite to entering the program, patients fill out a detailed questionnaire about their weight, medical and social history, and participate in a two-part evaluation interview. During the first interview, the questionnaire is reviewed with the patient, and any reported abnormality is discussed in detail. The interviewer explains the program at length to the patient. At the close of the interview, he issues a week's supply of food diary forms to fill out and arranges for a second interview with the patient and spouse or significant other. The food diary is reviewed during the second interview with the patient and spouse, and remaining questions about the program are answered. An assessment is made of the patient's motivation, ability to follow instructions, and ability to carry out a repetitive, boring task for a week (completion of a food diary). The program is reviewed with the patient and spouse who is asked to aid in the behavior change program by being available as a "student" to whom the patient can teach the weekly lesson. The evaluation costs $35.00 to $50.00, and the group treatment program costs $200 for ten weeks of instruction and ten weeks of maintenance. Twenty-five dollars is refunded if patients complete their homework. Patients are asked to pay all fees in advance.

Criteria for exclusion from group treatment are not rigid. We have eliminated people who were acutely psychotic, severely depressed, experiencing severe marital discord, unable to follow instructions, and illiterate, as well as patients who would rather have psychiatric help unrelated to weight loss.

Treatment Procedure

Treatment groups contain six to thirteen patients of mixed ages and sexes, a group leader, and a co-therapist who helps the leader weigh patients and check homework. The groups meet for one and a half hours each week. Patients are weighed in private at the weekly sessions. Each patient graphs his own weight change and the group average weight change for the previous week. This exercise provides feedback for each individual about his performance without encouraging him to compete directly with other patients (Figure 10-1).

The therapists check each patient's homework and determine his weekly contingent refund. Money is returned if the assignment for the week is completed. After weighing patients and checking their homework, new homework forms and an outline for the current lesson are distributed. The weekly lesson is presented in a didactic lecture style. Subsequent group discussion is guided by the leader who elicits and verbally reinforces examples of success. Discussion of emotional issues and personal problems is discouraged.

During the maintenance period, patients are asked to practice all of the techniques learned in the previous five weeks. Attendance at maintenance meetings is advised but optional. During these sessions, patients are weighed and any problems with the program are discussed with the therapist.

FIGURE 10-1

The patient and therapist each have a copy of the master data sheet. Each week, the patient records his weight, weight change, cumulative weight change, and the average weight change for the entire therapy group in the appropriate squares on the form. He plots his weight change and the group change for the previous week on the graph. This visual display gives the patient feedback about his progress and allows him to compare his performance with the group as a whole. In this example, the patient's weight change is shown by the dark line, the group mean change is shown by the light line. The shaded areas are maintenance or practice periods in the program.

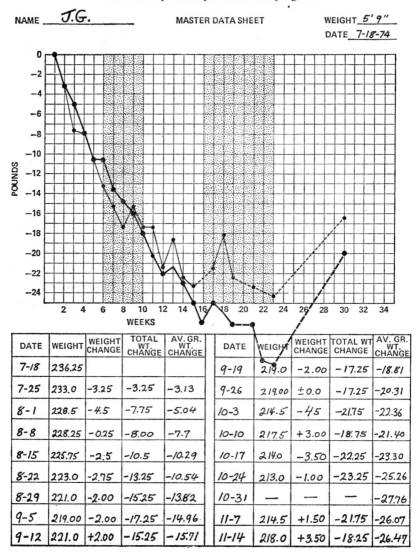

NAME __J.G.__   MASTER DATA SHEET   WEIGHT _5' 9"_

DATE _7-18-74_

DATE	WEIGHT	WEIGHT CHANGE	TOTAL WT. CHANGE	AV. GR. WT. CHANGE	DATE	WEIGHT	WEIGHT CHANGE	TOTAL WT CHANGE	AV. GR. WT. CHANGE
7-18	236.25				9-19	219.0	-2.00	-17.25	-18.81
7-25	233.0	-3.25	-3.25	-3.13	9-26	219.00	±0.0	-17.25	-20.31
8-1	228.5	-4.5	-7.75	-5.04	10-3	214.5	-4.5	-21.75	-22.36
8-8	228.25	-0.25	-8.00	-7.7	10-10	217.5	+3.00	-18.75	-21.40
8-15	225.75	-2.5	-10.5	-10.29	10-17	214.0	-3.50	-22.25	-23.30
8-22	223.0	-2.75	-13.25	-10.54	10-24	213.0	-1.00	-23.25	-25.26
8-29	221.0	-2.00	-15.25	-13.82	10-31	—	—	—	-27.76
9-5	219.00	-2.00	-17.25	-14.96	11-7	214.5	+1.50	-21.75	-26.07
9-12	221.0	+2.00	-15.25	-15.71	11-14	218.0	+3.50	-18.25	-26.47

TABLE 10-1

Combined data for all patients entering seven weight control groups. Each group received ten instruction sessions. The data in the Table were collected at visit 10 or the patient's final visit if he dropped out of the program. The figures in parentheses exclude patients who dropped out of the program prior to visit 10. Two patients who did not attend the final meeting are included in these figures.

Number of patients			Age	Mean		Range	
Female	50	(45)	Female	35	(37.2)	17-60	(20-60)
Male	12	(9)	Male	43.6	(42.5)	27-64	(27-64)
Total	62	(54)	Total	37.5	(37.4)	17-64	(20-64)

Starting weight			Mean		Range	
Female	209.6		(207.6)	140-358	(140-358)	
Male	258.8		(257.6)	· 196-318	(196-318)	
Total	218.8		(215.9)	140-358	(140-358)	

Percent losing weight			Percent losing over ten pounds		
Female	94%	(90%)	Female	40%	(42%)
Male	91%	(100%)	Male	42%	(55%)
Total	93%	(92.6%)	Total	40%	(44%)

Weight change		Mean	Range	
Female	—9.6	(—9.7)	—32.5 to +7.5	(—32.5 to +7.5)
Male	—10.0	(—12.2)	—27 to +3.0	(—27 to —1)
Total	—9.7	(—10.8)	—32.5 to +7.5	(—32.5 to +7.5)

Results

Sixty-two patients have been included in behavioral weight control groups. They have been distributed among seven groups. Four groups had ten weeks of instruction and one follow-up session approximately ten weeks after the final session. The final three groups had five weeks of instructions followed by five weeks of maintenance with optional weekly weighing at the Clinic, then an additional five weeks of instruction and a final five weeks of maintenance or practice.

A detailed summary of the data we have accumulated on these patients is shown in Table 10-1. Eighty percent of our patients have been women. The age of the patients has averaged 37.5 years old, with a range of 17 to 64 years of age. The patients' beginning weight has ranged from 140 to 358 pounds, with an average of 218.8 pounds. Ninety-three percent of the patients have lost some weight, and 40 percent have lost more than 10 pounds dur-

TABLE 10-2
Patients Dropping out of the Weight Control Program

Sex	Age	Onset	Last Visit	Weight Change	Reason
M	31	Adult	8	—1	Refused to come back, program not working
M	54	Adult .	4	—1¼	Repeating the course, not helped the second time
F	17	Child	5	—3	Post kidney transplant, on immunosuppressive drugs, no longer interested
F	48	Adult	8	—6½	Went on summer vacation
F	35	Child	3	+2	Post ileal bypass with poor result, severe marital discord
F	19	Adult	6	—18½	Losing well, feels no need for more lessons
M	55	Adult	5	—5¼	Out of town 4 weeks—sick following 4 weeks, received materials in mail
F	17	Child	7	—9	Didn't want to come back, no reason given

ing the ten weeks of instruction. The range of weight change recorded at the tenth treatment session has varied between a maximum loss of 32.5 pounds and a gain of 7.5 pounds. The average weight loss for these patients was 9.7 pounds. There is no statistically significant difference between the male and female patients on any of the measures of change. The dropout rate for the program is 13 percent (8 individuals). These patients quit the program at different sessions for idiosyncratic reasons (Table 10-2). When the age, baseline weight, and weight loss data are corrected for dropouts, no significant trends emerge (Table 10-3).

Follow-up has been for a short interval of 1-2 months following the tenth session. Only 53 percent of our patients have returned for follow-up. The average weight loss for this group during the ten-week program was 10.7 pounds. During the 1-2 month interval, after the group stopped meeting, the average group member who returned for follow-up lost an additional 1.2 pounds. One year follow-up is currently in progress.

TABLE 10-3

Weight Loss for Childhood and Adult Onset Obese Patients
(Figures in brackets exclude patients who dropped out of the program prior to visit 10)

Onset	N	Number losing weight	Number gaining weight	No weight change	Average weight change	Average beginning weight
Childhood	32 (29)	28 (27)	3 (2)	1 (0)	−9.25 (−9.51)	226.6 (225.0)
Adult	30 (25)	27 (22)	2 (2)	1 (1)	−10.1 (−10.75)	211.6 (205.2)

FIGURE 10-2

The cumulative average weight loss for seven behavioral weight control groups. The groups indicated by stars received ten weeks of instruction with a follow-up meeting 6-10 weeks after the final group session. For the purpose of illustration and comparison, all of the follow-up sessions are plotted at week 20. The groups indicated by squares received a program that alternated five weeks of instruction with five weeks of maintenance or practice. The solid lines represent periods of weekly instruction. The broken lines represent periods of maintenance or follow-up.

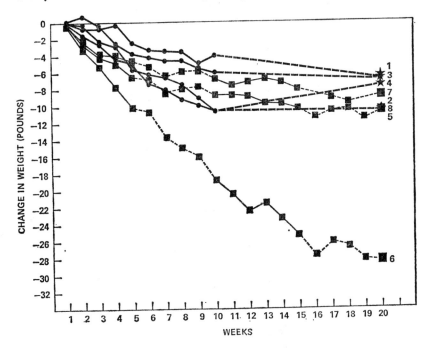

The groups have included 32 childhood onset (before 10 years old) and 30 adult onset overweight individuals. Table 10-3 shows the data for these two groups of patients. Although adult onset obese patients tended to be lighter initially and lose slightly more weight in the program, these differences are not statistically significant.

A graph of the weekly average weight loss for each group shows a marked difference between groups (Figure 10-2). The group composition and non-specific therapeutic effects appear to

FIGURE 10-3

Individual cumulative weight change for Group 6. The shaded areas are periods of maintenance or practice. The solid lines represent periods of consecutive weekly attendance. The dashed lines represent periods of interrupted attendance.

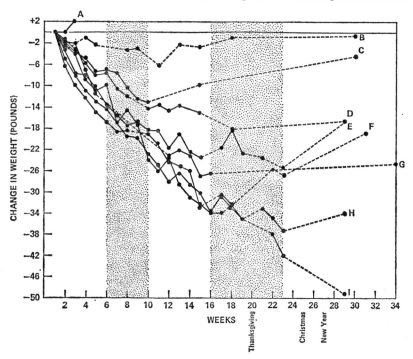

be important variables in determining group outcome. These variables include leadership style, leader interest in the program, and leader experience with the program. The author of the weekly lessons, who had both the greatest familiarity with their content and the greatest vested interest in their success, obtained the best results.

Figure 10-2 also compares two different program formats. The groups numbered 1, 2, 3, 4 had ten continuous weeks of instruction. Their end point and follow-up average weight are marked by a star on the graph. The groups labeled 6, 7, 8 were given the program in alternating five-week periods of instruction and practice. Despite greater therapeutic contact, there does not appear to

FIGURE 10-4

The average cumulative weight change for a group receiving 20 behavioral sessions. "F" indicates a follow-up session one month after session 10 and one month before session 11. "V" indicates a break of two months for summer vacation. The broken line represents an interruption in the program.

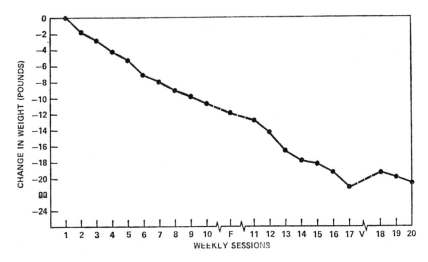

be a significantly greater amount of weight loss with the latter format. Unfortunately, the patients returning for follow-up are a biased sample of group members, and definite conclusions cannot be reached about the program format from these data.

A weekly plot of weight change for individuals within a single group shows a widely differing therapeutic effect (Figure 10-3). Patients who respond poorly are identifiable by the fourth week. These individuals continue to do poorly for a variety of reasons. An analysis of patient food diaries and homework indicates many of them do not follow the instructions or use only the techniques they feel are most valuable or least onerous. The patients represented in Figure 10-3 demonstrate several other apparent predictors of failure. Patient A was in the midst of a difficult marital situation when the group began. Patient B is a successful businessman who could not attend many of the group sessions. Patient C had her weight loss interrupted by a five-week trip to Japan. The maintenance period for this group included Thanksgiving, Christ-

FIGURE 10-5

Individual cumulative weight change for the group shown in Figure 4. "F" indicates a follow-up session one month after session 10 and one month before session 11. "V" indicates a break of two months for summer vacation. The broken line represents an interruption in the program.

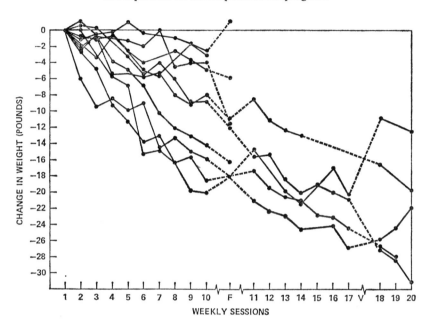

mas, and New Year's Day. Despite some gain of weight during the holidays, many patients indicated amazement at their relative success at maintenance during these periods of traditional feasting.

The Stanford program has been designed to cover a total of forty weeks. This includes twenty prepared lessons and twenty weeks of interspersed maintenance or practice. One group has completed the entire sequence (Figure 10-4). Their weight loss continued while the groups continued to meet, but slowed when weekly contact with the group was interrupted. The period between session 10 and F (follow-up) is one month. Between F and session 11 is also one month. V represents a two-month break for summer vacation. This plot suggests that at least part of the

FIGURE 10-6

Cumulative weight loss in three consecutive behavioral weight control groups led by three different therapists using the same written program. The shaded area represents the five-week maintenance periods.

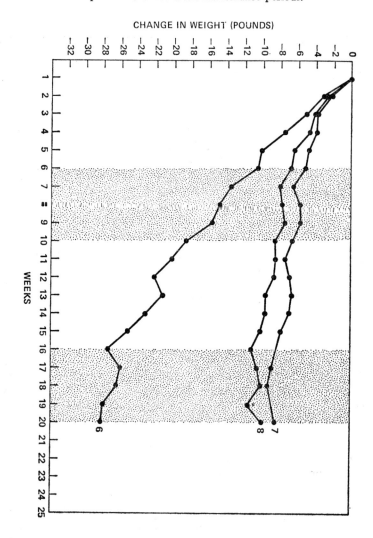

effect of the behavior modification can be attributed to either group contact or to the presence of the therapist.

Figure 10-5 is a plot of the individual patients included in Figure 10-4. A strong selection for success is indicated by these data. Those who lose weight during the first ten weeks of instruction are willing to pay additional money to maintain contact with the group for an additional ten weeks.

Discussion

The program we have developed is an empirical approach to the behavioral control of weight. An analysis of the data shows a large difference in individual patient response to the program and a difference between groups of patients led by different therapists. A comparison of group outcome data (Figure 10-6) suggests that these unaccounted-for variables may be more potent than the "behavior modification" *per se.*

Mahoney and others (Mahoney, 1975a, 1975b; Jordan and Levitz, 1975) have discussed some of the theoretical issues relevant to the behavioral treatment of obesity: overweight individuals may not differ from their thin counterparts in actual eating behaviors; the behavioral changes we claim result from the behavioral intervention in this type of program may not actually occur; and obesity may have non-learned elements that we cannot affect by behavior modification techniques. All of these points can be raised when attempting to interpret our results.

This clinical program to treat obesity lacks much of the theoretical and experimental elegance needed to adequately address these issues. The reasons for our limited success can probably be found both in the techniques used and the structure the program provides for a therapist to exert non-specific but powerful effect on his patients.

Chapter 11

A Clinical and Research Questionnaire for Obese Patients

W. Stewart Agras, James M. Ferguson, Charles Greaves, Brandon Qualls, Colleen S. W. Rand, Janet Ruby, Albert J. Stunkard, C. Barr Taylor, Joellen Werne, and Carolyn Wright

A university-based eating disorders clinic is in a position to fulfill several roles. These can be summarized under the division of service, research, and teaching. To facilitate research in our clinical or service program, we have developed a questionnaire to systematically collect information about our patient population. This list of questions includes standard medical, demographic, and sociologic items. Most of the questions are "closed ended" or easily adaptable for rapid data analysis.

Patients receive a copy of the questionaire if they express interest in the behavioral weight control program when they call the clinic. Only patients who return the questionnaire are called for subsequent evaluation interviews. Most of the forms are returned to the clinic with all items answered. The information received is reviewed with the patient during his evaluation interviews, and any medical or psychological abnormality reported by the patient is discussed at length. The questionnaire is then stored for subsequent data analysis.

This research was supported in part by the National Institute of Mental Health grant—MH 25568-01 for the Clinical and Experimental Study of Human Obesity.

TABLE 11-1

(Based on 12 Months)

Contacts: clinic phone, and other	Questionnaires distributed	Questionnaires returned	Patients retained
374	168	101	87

The response of patients to the questionnaire is shown in Table 11-1. The high rate of retention of patients returning the completed questionnaire indicates a significant screening value in addition to its primary purpose of data collection.

We are publishing this questionnaire to make it available for use *in toto* or as a tested model for anyone with a clinical or research interest in obesity. The final questions, order, and wording of the questionnaire represent a collaborative effort of the entire Stanford Eating Disorders Clinic staff. The authors are listed alphabetically.

STANFORD EATING DISORDERS CLINIC

QUESTIONNAIRE

Name:_____ Sex: M F   Age:_____ Birthdate:_____

Address:_____ Home phone:_____

_____ Office phone:_____

WEIGHT HISTORY:

1. Your present weight_____height_____

2. How would you describe your present weight? (circle one)

very　　　　　　slightly　　　　about
overweight　　　overweight　　　average

3. At what weight have you _felt_ your best or do you think you would feel your best?

_____

4. How much weight would you like to lose?_____

5. How dissatisfied are you with the way you look at this weight? (circle one)

Completely　　Moderately　　Neutral　　Moderately　　　Very
Satisfied　　　Satisfied　　　　　　　　Dissatisfied　　Dissatisfied

6. Do other people react to your weight problem? Yes___ No___ If yes, how do they react?

_____

_____

7. Why do you want to lose weight at this time?_____

_____

8. What are the attitudes of the following people about your attempt(s) to lose weight?

	Negative (e.g., disapprove, resentful)	Indifferent (e.g., don't care, don't help)	Positive (e.g., encourage, understanding)
Husband			
Wife			
Children			
Parents			
Employer			
Friends			

9. Do the attitudes or behavior of your spouse or children affect your weight loss or gain? Yes___ No___ If yes, please describe:_____

_____

_____

10. Indicate the periods in your life when you have been overweight on the following table. Where appropriate, list your maximum weight for each period and number of pounds you were overweight. Briefly describe any methods you used to lose weight, e.g., diet, shots, pills, in that five-year episode. Also list any significant life events you feel were related to either your weight gain or loss, e.g., college tests, marriage, pregnancies, illness.

Age	Maximum Weight	# Pounds Overweight	Methods Used to Lose Weight	Significant Events Related to Weight Change
Birth				
0 - 5				
5 - 10				
10 - 15				
15 - 20				
20 - 25				
25 - 30				
30 - 35				
35 - 40				
40 - 45				
45 - 50				
50 - 55				
55 - 60				
60 - 65				

11. How do you feel your weight affects your daily activities? (circle one)

   No effect   Some effect   Often interferes   Extreme effect

12. How physically active are you? (circle one)

   Very active   Active   Average   Inactive   Very inactive

13. What do you do for physical exercise and how often do you do it?•

FREQUENCY (daily, weekly, monthly)	ACTIVITY (swiming, jogging, dancing)

14. A number of different ways of losing weight are listed below. Please indicate which methods you have used by filling the appropriate blanks.

	Ages Used	Number of Times Used	Max.Wt. Lost	Comments: Length of time weight loss maintained; success; difficulties
TOPS				
Weight Watchers				
HCG shots				
Pills				
Supervised diet				
Unsupervised diet				
Starvation diet				
Behavior mod				
Psychotherapy				
Hypnosis				
Other				

15. Which method did you use for the longest period of time?_____

16. In your attempts to lose weight, have you ever had a physical or emotional reaction of such severity that it impaired your family and/or work relationships or functioning?

   Yes___ No___ If yes, please describe the symptoms and how long they lasted.

_____

_____

_____

17. Have you had a major mood change after a significant weight loss?

    Yes___ No___ If yes, indicate on the following checklist those changes:

	Not at All	A Little Bit	Moderately	Quite a Bit	Extremely
a. Depressed, sad, feeling down or unhappy?					
b. Feeling anxious, nervous or restless?					
c. Feeling weak?					
d. Feeling elated?					
e. Feeling easily irritated, annoyed or angry?					
f. Feeling fatigued, worn out?					
g. Being preoccupied with food and eating?					
h. Feeling a lack of self-confidence?					

18. What usually goes wrong with your weight loss programs? _____

_____

_____

_____

MEDICAL HISTORY:

19. What are your present medical problems? _____

_____

_____

20. What medications or drugs are you taking? _____

_____

_____

21. Are you allergic to medications, drugs or foods? _____

_____

22. Please list any hospitalization or operations. Indicate your age for each hospital admission.

    Age   Reason for hospitalization

_____   _____

_____   _____

_____   _____

_____   _____

23. Please list, by age, any serious illnesses you have had which have not required hospitalization or operations:

   Age   Illness

   _____   _____

   _____   _____

   _____   _____

   _____   _____

. 24. Please describe any medical problems you have which are complicated by your weight.

   _____

   _____

   _____

   _____

25. When did you last have a complete physical examination?_____

26. Who is your current doctor?_____

27. How much alcohol do you usually drink per week?_____

28. Please list any psychiatric contact, individual counseling, or marital counseling that you have had or are now having.

   Age   Reason for contact and type of therapy

   _____   _____

   _____   _____

   _____   _____

SOCIAL HISTORY:

29. Please describe your present occupation_____

   _____

30. How long have you worked for your present employer?_____

31. Circle the last year of school attended:

   1 2 3 4 5 6 7 8   9 10 11 12   1 2 3 4   M.A.   Ph.D.   Other_____
   Grade School   High School   College

32. Present marital status: (circle one)

   Single   Married   Divorced   Widowed   Separated   Engaged

33. Please answer the following questions for each marriage:

   Date of marriage   _____ _____ _____

   Date of termination   _____ _____ _____

   Reason (death, divorce, etc.) _____ _____ _____

   Number of children   _____ _____ _____

34. Please describe your present spouse's occupation in detail_____

_____

35. Spouse's age_____ Weight_____ Height_____

36. How would you describe your spouse's weight? (circle one)

<table>
<tr><td>very
overweight</td><td>slightly
overweight</td><td>about
average</td><td>slightly
underweight</td><td>very
underweight</td></tr>
</table>

37. Please list your children's age, sex, height, weight, and circle whether they are overweight, average, or underweight. Include any children from previous marriages whether they are living with you or not.

Age	Sex	Weight	Height	Overweight		Average	Underweight	
____	___	_____	_____	very	slightly	average	slightly	very
____	___	_____	_____	very	slightly	average	slightly	very
____	___	_____	_____	very	slightly	average	slightly	very
____	___	_____	_____	very	slightly	average	slightly	very
____	___	_____	_____	very	slightly	average	slightly	very

38. Who lives in your house with you?_____

_____

39. Is your father living? Yes___ No___ Father's age now or age and cause of death___

_____

40. Is your mother living? Yes___ No___ Mother's age now or age and cause of death___

_____

41. Describe your father's occupation_____

42. Describe your mother's occupation_____

43. Describe your father's weight while you were growing up: (circle one)

<table>
<tr><td>very
overweight</td><td>slightly
overweight</td><td>about
average</td><td>slightly
underweight</td><td>very
underweight</td></tr>
</table>

44. Describe your mother's weight while you were growing up: (circle one)

<table>
<tr><td>very
overweight</td><td>slightly
overweight</td><td>about
average</td><td>slightly
underweight</td><td>very
underweight</td></tr>
</table>

45. Please describe your family attitudes toward food and eating while you were growing up

_____

_____

_____

46. Were your parents ever separated or divorced? Yes___ No___ If yes, how old were you?_____

47. Who raised you as a child?_____

48. What was your relationship with your father like? (circle one)

    Excellent   Good   Average   Below average   Poor

49. What was your relationship with your mother like? (circle one)

    Excellent   Good   Average   Below average   Poor

50. Please list your brothers' and sisters' ages, sex, present weight, height, and circle whether they are overweight, average, or underweight.

Age	Sex	Weight	Height	Overweight		Average	Underweight	
____	___	_____	_____	very	slightly	average	slightly	very
____	___	_____	_____	very	slightly	average	slightly	very
____	___	_____	_____	very	slightly	average	slightly	very
____	___	_____	_____	very	slightly	average	slightly	very

51. Please write any other information you feel is relevant to your weight problem below. This would include interactions with your family and friends that might sabotage a weight loss program, or any part of your family history that is related and/or relevant to your weight problem.

_____

_____

_____

_____

_____

_____

_____

_____

_____

_____

_____

_____

_____

_____

_____

_____

Chapter 12

Affective and Cognitive Behavior Change: Essential Components to Comprehensive Obesity Treatment

Gerard J. Musante

Results of behavior modification have sparked renewed enthusiasm in the field of obesity treatment. The work of Stuart (1967, 1971) and others (Penick, Filion, Fox, and Stunkard, 1971; Wollersheim, 1970) demonstrates the fruitfulness of this approach. Behavioral treatment of obesity, however, is in an early stage of development. While enthusiasm may be well founded, results thus far are still tentative and not conclusive. For example, many reports have been conducted with a very carefully selected volunteer population of college students (Hagen, 1974; Harris, 1969). Many aspects of behavioral treatment need to be reevaluated and extended. Weight losses have not been large enough in absolute terms to demonstrate clinical utility. Long term follow-up has been provided in only a few cases. While Stuart (1967, 1971) and Penick et al. (1971) report excellent results, their clinical populations are small. Only one report (Musante, 1975) replicates results of the magnitude achieved by these two researchers with a large group of severely obese patients.

Unfortunately, behavioral treatment continues to be primarily a repetition of Ferster's (Ferster, Nurnberger, and Levitt, 1962) and Stuart's (1967) operant techniques. The behavioral approach to obesity treatment is in danger of being reduced to lists of stimulus and environmental control procedures, such as, "Chew food 20 times; knives and forks down after each bite; shop from a list." Such lists excite the less informed but may cause necessary research to be stopped if what is expected does not occur. Operant techniques alone may be insufficient. Specific environmental control techniques may not be generalizable to any given situation in view of a lack of large weight losses in the behavioral literature. Little attention has been given to affective and cognitive re-education, which may be essential components for long-lasting behavior change. It is possible that the excellent results reported by Stuart (1967, 1971) were in part a result of the individual treatment, allowing Stuart to attend to cognitive and affective behavior to a greater extent than is actually reported.

This chapter offers an explanation of why previous behavioral treatments may be incomplete, and suggests procedures for comprehensive treatment including affective and cognitive behavior change techniques. Suggestions are based on clinical experience with over 1000 obese patients of the Dietary Rehabilitation Clinic, a multi-modal outpatient program at Duke University Medical Center.

Description of the Dietary Rehabilitation Clinic

The Dietary Rehabilitation Clinic (DRC) serves the refractory obese patient, the veteran of every type of weight loss program. No pre-selection or screening factors are used. Self-selection does occur on the basis of patients coming to Duke as a last resort, and secondarily by the financial ability to leave home and come to a private clinic. DRC patients come from all over the country to participate at Duke. They eat 3 dietary meals a day, 7 days a week, in the Clinic Dining Room. Patients are not hospitalized but are on their own recognizance while in Durham. Though it is an outpatient program, it is intensive in nature. Treatment includes daily weigh-in, with brief consultation available with a physician, behavioral psychologist, and dietitian, prepared meals, medical supervision, weekly behavior therapy groups, and a lecture series. A more complete description of specific procedures has been published elsewhere (Musante, in press).

The DRC program provides an intensive view of the behavior of obese patients. Eating behavior as well as socialization, and day-to-day cognitive and affective behaviors can be monitored. As a result of such experience, the DRC program has undergone a series of developmental changes. It began solely as a dietary program. It grew into a program emphasizing behavioral control of eating. DRC is now a more comprehensive program and includes behavioral approaches to diet construction and management, medical care delivery, time and activity management, and cognitive and affective treatments to change aspects of behavior. It is felt that these are necessary components of effective treatment.

Theoretical Framework

There are numerous theories of the etiology and dynamics of obesity. The traditional concept is that personality disturbance precipitates overeating, and obesity is a symptom of this underlying disturbance. Since personality factors trigger inappropriate eating in this theory, intervention is aimed at changing personality.

A behavioral analysis of obesity, as delineated by Stuart (1971), views inappropriate behavior as the initial step in the chain, however. For example (from Stuart, 1971):

BEHAVIOR——>CONSEQUENCES——>THOUGHTS; FEELINGS

e.g.

underexercising by double }
parking in front of store }——>weight gain——> e.g. depression

According to this conception, it is the obese state itself which precipitates the thoughts and feelings associated with personality problems. "The behavioral approach intervenes by attempting to change the individual's eating patterns so that he can have different experiences in the world, these experiences leading in turn to changes in the thoughts and feelings which comprise the messages which he gives himself" (Stuart, 1971, p. 44).

This conception is correct insofar as it goes. As Stuart himself points out, the consequences, that is weight loss, increased mobility, and social acceptance, and changes in thoughts and feelings are often delayed because people need to lose large amounts of weight, which takes time. Sometimes the overeater is faced with the impossible burden of giving up his pleasure in eating while having to wait months or years before he finds alternate satisfactions. Therefore, intervention at only the first step in this chain (Behavior) is not powerful enough. Massive weight loss achieved in very short periods of time through hospitalized fasting has proven to be insufficient motivation to control weight (Swanson and Dinello, 1970). Essentially, eating behavior remains the same. Intervention only at the third point (Thoughts and Feelings) also is not enough, as demonstrated by the lack of positive results achieved by traditional psychotherapy in the treatment of obesity.

It appears that attacking the problem simultaneously at all three points is a necessary treatment strategy. Instead of Stuart's linear approach, a more efficient model may be a circular approach.

A conception of the etiology of obesity and the model for treatment at DRC is:

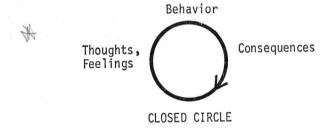

We know that any problematic behavior has certain negative consequences. These consequences produce a negative affective and cognitive component which some may conceptualize as personality. This negative affect or cognition is a stimulus for pre-potent behavior—in this case, for eating and inactivity. Of course, this behavioral response produces similar negative consequences. The circle is thus completed and also begun. There is no need for the model, furthermore, to look for a beginning point in this process, since it is a self-generated process. The closed circle of obesity necessitates treatment which breaks the chain at all three points.

Stuart (1967) suggests that the feeling of self-control gained from successful small steps of controlling eating behavior will provide sufficient reinforcement to continue the treatment. What is suggested here, however, is that patients need other reinforcement if they are to continue, i.e., significant rapid weight loss and positive changes in affective and cognitive states must be part of the treatment, as well as instruction in overt behavior change.

Treatment

At DRC the goal is to intervene at all three points. This is done by applying behavior principles to as many aspects of treatment as possible—the diet, the medical and behavioral care, the patient-doctor relationship—thereby emphasizing cognitive, affective, and motoric reconditioning.

Behavioral Approach to Diet Construction

Studies emphasizing the behavioral control of eating have for the most part not dealt with the issue of diet, nutrition, or the affective and cognitive components related to it. Many studies instruct no specific dietary limitation (Harris, 1969; Stuart, 1967), while others simply encourage patients to reduce caloric intake or follow a sensible diet (Wollersheim, 1960; Harris and Hallbauer, 1973; Harris and Bruner, 1969). Stuart (1971) was the first behaviorist to include food management as a necessity and suggest the use of a food exchange list, which is not adaptable to social pressures or the psychological stresses of hunger. At DRC we observed that the psychological stresses of hunger, as well as eccentric food gathering and eating behavior common to the obese and food-deprived person, may result not from the number of calories allowed but rather how menus are constructed and the affective and cognitive approach to food. We observed that when patients, particularly new patients at DRC, are served 700 calories per day in pre-planned menus, they report satisfaction and seldom feel hungry. When new patients are allowed to construct their own meals from a list of menus, they seem confused as if a stimulus overload had occurred. When many cues occur and too many choices are available, patients begin to exhibit the following behaviors.

1. Rising anxiety.
2. Rumination about food.
3. Over-stressing of calories—asking for 10 calories worth of onions or cottage cheese to reach their "quota" for the day.
4. Skipping or scrimping at breakfast and lunch to be able to add on at dinner.
5. Requesting large amounts of one or two low calorie foods, and then habituating to large portions.
6. Overdoing spices and condiments.
7. Trying a little of everything and making up unusual combinations to fit into the caloric allotment, likened to nibbling from the refrigerator.
8. Complaining that eating slowly makes food cold.
9. Overemphasizing smell and taste of food.

Patients need to be taught slowly to construct menus. This behavior must be shaped. While the content of the diet may be an insignificant factor in weight control (Bray, 1970), menu planning must be thought of as an important part of the treatment. Prepared menus which specify the desired target behavior in small steps provide a goal and give patients *in vivo* experience with what constitutes appropriate foods and portions. Stimulus overload and overconcern with "the diet" is minimized in this way and is an important step toward correcting misconceptions concerning the emphasis most patients have on diet content.

A suggested shaping of dieting behavior can be initiated by new patients remaining on a fixed menu plan, with substitutions only for sound medical reasons. Level I treatment can be a weekly menu plan of 3 different menus a day, 4 different menus for the month. Such an experience would alleviate decision making for which patients may not be ready. It would help the affective state of the patients to reduce anxiety concerning food and selection of food. Practice with what constitutes appropriate portions is important. Supplemental videotapes and other materials on nutrition can be made available. On Level I, patients also should begin to use a diary by entering what they will eat *prior* to having their meals.

Level II patients may make some substitutions. The self-selection process can begin here. Diaries can be checked periodically to see how their learning is progressing. Level II patients may construct their own pre-planned menus. As they progress on the program, all the foods are common to increase probability of generalization. These patients can practice preparing menus and corresponding shopping lists.

In addition, cognitive components relating to food must be changed. For example, rather than having patients devise "low calorie desserts," we teach that a meal is an appropriate portion of specific foods—and that dessert is *not* part of a meal. Also, the excessive use of seasonings and spices is discouraged. The taste and appeal of food is de-emphasized. "We eat to live not live to eat" is the cognitive change that is sought.

One important procedure for changing cognitions and affect is verbal reconditioning. Obese patients are typically self-denigrating. They talk about and think about themselves in a negative manner, and are in the habit of attaching moral significance to their eating behavior. If a patient adheres to his diet, he describes this behavior as "being good today." Departure from the diet is accompanied by feelings of guilt and failure, and is referred to as being bad or "cheating." At DRC we concentrate on extinguishing negative verbal behavior and reinforcing positive verbal behavior. Non-adherence to the diet is referred to as "unstructured eating" rather than cheating, a term which helps remove moral connotations.

Behavioral Approach to the Patient-Doctor Relationship

DRC patients often suffer concomitant medical problems, and these are followed by the physician on the program. Through a complete physical and medical work-up, the misconception that they are "made differently" or that physical abnormalities are the cause of their problem is changed. Such cognitive re-education is reinforced at check-in during didactic lectures on medical topics related to obesity. Also, how a physician "talks" to an overweight patient can have a major effect on the course of treatment. What do you say when a patient is discouraged about not losing "fast enough"? How do you respond when a patient does not want to weigh every morning any more? What can be said to a patient who has been structured, but *gains* weight the next day? What do you say to a patient who has been on a plateau for 10 days? What do you tell a patient if he or she requests a diuretic? How do you react when a patient tells you he has been unstructured? These are crucial questions in the patient-doctor relationship. How a physician responds to his patient can determine whether the cognitive and affective qualities of the patient are altered. Improper responses on the part of the physician can otherwise reinforce the maladaptive behavior of the patient. The traditional doctor-patient relationship whereby the doctor is the active authority while the patient passively receives treatment and is the participant is not valid in the case of obesity treatment. Here, the patient is the active participant. Dieting is a negative therapy, while almost everything else that doctors do involves something positive (Feinstein, 1974). This cognitive set of dependence and passivity must be altered, and requires behavioral changes on the part of both physician and patient.

Various treatment procedures also have subtle cognitive and affective components which must be considered. Daily weigh-in can be a critical experience for the obese individual. Obese individuals can have great anxiety about scales. Many actually fear seeing the numbers. If one goal is habituating daily weighing, the individual must deal with anxiety. Reduction of the anxiety can be accomplished by flooding—making patients stay on the scale for 5 minutes.

Behavioral Techniques

DRC treatment includes all elements typically reported concerning the behavioral control of eating. Stimulus control procedures are practiced in the dining room. Environmental control procedures are illustrated and discussed in the weekly behavior therapy groups. In addition, an emphasis is placed on cognitive change. Re-education, done in various ways, orientation procedures, daily check-in, didactic lectures, video-tapes, programmed learning packets, behavior therapy groups all provide repetition and reinforcement via different modalities. People learn in different ways at different rates.

Experience with large numbers of patients in this clinical setting has shown that people begin treatment with different levels of knowledge, sets, expectations. Some immediately work well within the behavioral framework while others take longer to accept ideas, change attitudes, change behavior, and initiate environmental planning techniques. Cognitive reconditioning procedures are leveled from beginners to advanced, with patients progressing at their own rate and receiving instruction via different modalities.

It is up to the patient to put behavioral practices into operation. This behavior is more likely to occur if he has a positive set, understands the practices, uses the behavioral vocabulary and is reinforced for positive verbal behavior.

Assertive training is an integral part of DRC treatment. The counterconditioning procedures of assertive training are included as a means by which patients develop a repertoire of assertive behavior rather than avoidance by overeating when they encounter high arousal situations associated with eating. Assertive training provides a systematic procedure for increasing the likelihood of social reinforcement, and provides the obese with an effective set of behaviors generalizable to a wide variety of situations. Unlike social pressure groups (i.e., TOPS), which provide social reinforcement for losing a certain number of pounds, reinforcement here occurs for positive changes in verbal, affective, and motoric behavior.

The aim of DRC is to develop an intensive treatment for obesity that can be used as a model for other programs. Protocols, techniques, and packages are being developed with the knowledge obtained in this intensive program for use on an outpatient group clinic basis and in the office of the private physician.

Chapter 13

Diet Modification in the Community

John P. Foreyt, Lynne W. Scott, and Antonio M. Gotto, Jr.

Cardiovascular diseases are the leading causes of death in the United States. The latest estimates indicate that more than 27 million persons in this country are afflicted with some form of cardiovascular disease (American Heart Association, 1974). Over one million deaths (about 54 percent of all deaths) each year are due to these diseases. Heart attack is the leading killer. Almost 4 million Americans have a history of heart attack and/or angina pectoris. In 1971, it claimed 675,580 lives (National Center for Health Statistics, 1974).

The estimated economic costs to this country for 1974 were staggering: $8.6 billion in lost wages; $6.8 billion in hospital and nursing home services; $2.6 billion in physician and nursing services; $1.1 billion in research and construction; and $0.6 billion in cost of medication, for a total cost of $19.7 billion dollars (National Center for Health Statistics, 1974). Add to this figure costs that are difficult to measure, such as losses in management skills, production knowledge, personnel training and development, and labor turnover and one begins to see the scope of the problem.

The United States is not alone in this problem. All of the in-

This work was supported by Grant No. HL17269 from the National Heart and Lung Institute for the National Research and Demonstration Center.

dustrialized countries in the world are being ravaged by this epidemic. Finland leads the world in mortality rates for males due to heart disease, followed by the United States, Scotland, Australia, Canada, New Zealand, England and Wales, Norway, Denmark, Austria, the Netherlands, Sweden, Switzerland, and Italy, in that order (Stamler, 1973). Men are most vulnerable, but women tend to catch up with men after menopause.

Serious attempts to control this epidemic are just beginning. The overall approach being taken is a strategy emphasizing *primary prevention* of heart disease through control of the major coronary risk factors.

RISK FACTORS

The term, risk factor, refers to habits, traits, and abnormalities associated with a 100 percent or more increase in susceptibility to heart disease (Stamler, 1973), i.e., the presence of risk factors indicates a greater proneness to the premature onset of the disease. Many research studies (e.g., Chapman and Massey, 1964; Dawber, Kannel and McNamara, 1964; Dawber, Kannel, Revotskie, and Kagen, 1962; Kannel, Castelli, Gordon, and McNamara, 1971) conducted over the last several decades have demonstrated an association between certain factors and the development of coronary heart disease. As mentioned in Chapter 7, these risk factors include:

1. Elevated level of serum cholesterol
2. Elevated blood pressure
3. Cigarette smoking
4. Obesity
5. Elevated level of serum triglycerides
6. Heredity
7. Diabetes
8. Overweight
9. Diet high in saturated fats
10. Lack of exercise
11. Personality type A

About 80 percent of the people in the United States who die or are disabled by coronary heart disease have one or more of the first three risk factors (Task Force on Arteriosclerosis of the National Heart and Lung Institute, 1971):

1. Elevated serum cholesterol 2. Elevated blood pressure
3. Cigarette smoking

In males between ages 30 and 49 the risk of coronary heart disease is 5 times higher for those with serum cholesterol levels above 260 mg per 100 ml than for those with values below 220 mg per 100 ml (Dawber et al., 1962).

What we need to determine are the most effective approaches for combating coronary heart disease through the control of the major risk factors.

OVERWEIGHT

Researchers using behavior modification techniques have reported some success in dealing with one of the risk factors, overweight. By viewing overweight as primarily a function of poor food-related habits, behavior modifiers have developed a fairly large number of techniques, broadly based on learning principles, aimed at helping overweight persons achieve control over their eating by manipulating both the antecedent and consequent conditions of their behavior. This line of research has advanced our knowledge of overweight and its treatment, and some of these techniques seem to help many who have previously been unable to control their weight.

These behavioral techniques to achieve weight loss have become extremely popular today for several reasons. First, traditional treatments of obesity haven't had much success in dealing with the problem. Stunkard's (1958, p. 79) widely quoted statement summarizing his review of the results of traditional approaches to obesity, "Most obese persons will not stay in treatment for obesity. Of those who stay in treatment, most will not lose weight, and of those who do lose weight, most will regain it" seems to be as true today as it was when he said it in 1958. Second, behavioral techniques have become popular because weight reduction offers an excellent opportunity for behavior therapists to test theoretical issues while still maintaining clinical relevance. Many basic research issues can be investigated without resort to analogue studies of trivial problems, such as snake and spider phobias, so popular during the 1960's, in the systematic desensitization literature. And third, being a risk factor associated with cardiovascular diseases, overweight is clearly a major problem in our society.

There are two major procedural lines of behavioral research in treating overweight. One evolved from the classical conditioning paradigm and attempts to create conditioned aversion responses to certain foods. This approach has been fairly popular with other addictive, compulsive, and persistent behavior disorders, especially alcoholism (Rachman and Teasdale, 1969) and the sexual deviations (Feldman and MacCulloch, 1971). Aversion therapy consists of a number of techniques in which the conditioned stimulus (actual food, pictures of food, the individual engaging in eating behavior, or the imagery of food or food related behaviors) is repeatedly followed by some aversive unconditioned stimulus (electric shock, bad odor, chemical nauseant, or the imagery of unpleasant scenes).

The rationale for using such techniques in treating overeating is that the learned avoidance of certain foods will result in reduced caloric intake, and eventually result in weight loss. Overall, this line of research has not produced very impressive results (Foreyt and Kennedy, 1971; Frohwirth, 1974; Kennedy and Foreyt, 1968; Meyer and Crisp, 1964; Thorpe, Schmidt, Brown, and Castell, 1964; Wijesinghe, 1973), and most investigators view them as possibly helpful only when used in combination with other methods.

The other, more popular, approach to treating overweight has come from the operant conditioning learning paradigm. These techniques are aimed at teaching individuals how to develop "self-control" over their food-related behaviors, and include self-monitoring (weight, food intake, and activity), environmental planning (control over the stimulus conditions surrounding eating behaviors), and behavioral programming (contingency contracts, token economies, self-rewards, and self-punishments) strategies. The results of these "self-control" procedures have been generally encouraging. Weight losses of about 1 to 2 pounds per week, which is the aim of these approaches, are not uncommon during treatment, and at the present time it apears that these approaches (e.g., Hagen, 1974; Penick, Filion, Fox, and Stunkard, 1971;

Stuart, 1967, 1971; Stuart and Davis, 1972) have been relatively successful in comparison to other treatments in producing short-term weight loss. More definitive conclusions must await five and ten year follow-up periods.

All of the behavioral techniques seem to work with some individuals, at least in producing initial weight losses. The most helpful behavioral approach for treating obesity seems to involve a combination of the following:

1. Self-control techniques for habit change
2. Nutritional information
3. Regular exercise program

Combining self-control techniques (along with therapist-reinforcement techniques, such as monetary contracts, to insure participation) with nutritional information and a regular exercise regimen should result in maximal weight reduction and its maintenance over a long-term period.

Many manuals and books which incorporate some of these techniques are available, including manuals by Hagen (Hagen, Wollersheim, and Paul, 1969), Jeffrey and colleagues (Christensen, Jeffrey, and Pappas, 1973; Mahoney and Jeffrey, 1974), and McReynolds and colleagues (Paulsen, McReynolds, Lutz, and Kohrs, 1974). These manuals, along with the book by Stuart and Davis (1972) *Slim Chance in a Fat World: Behavioral Control of Obesity*, can be very helpful in developing a treatment program for treating obesity.

With the many advances that have been made, there are still major problems (Foreyt, in press) in the research to date, including:

1. Lack of adequate follow-up periods, i.e., more than 1 year.
2. Presence of uncontrolled variables, i.e., the difficulty in attributing behavioral changes and weight losses to the behavioral treatments because of the presence of uncontrolled or poorly controlled variables during treatment.
3. Inability to generalize results, i.e., many studies have been done with mildly overweight college sophomore females.
4. Failure to report attrition data, i.e., many studies do not report what happens to the subjects who drop out of the program before completing it.

5. Lack of standards for reporting results, i.e., the many ways researchers report their data make comparisons among studies extremely difficult.
6. Difficulty in determining effective treatment components, i.e., since most treatment programs use a combination of techniques, it is difficult to determine the relative effectiveness of each component of the program.

The results of the research to date have generally shown the behavioral treatments to be superior to other forms of treatment, at least during reported short-term follow-up periods. There is a guarded optimism among many therapists that further significant advances will be made in the next four years and that one of the risk factors of heart disease, overweight, may be at least treatable through behavioral approaches.

The question, "Can *other* risk factors leading to cardiovascular disease also be attacked through behavioral approaches?" still remains to be tested. Specifically, "Can one of the *major* risk factors, elevated lipids (serum cholesterol and triglycerides) be treated and reduced using behavioral techniques?"

THE BAYLOR DIET MODIFICATION PROGRAM

The Baylor Diet Modification Program is an attempt to do just that, attack one of the other risk factors, in this case, serum cholesterol and triglycerides, using behavioral techniques. The program is one of several projects which make up the National Heart and Blood Vessel Research and Demonstration Center. The Center, located at Baylor College of Medicine, Houston, is funded by a five-year grant from the National Heart and Lung Institute (NHLI) of the National Institutes of Health (NIH). The Director is Dr. Michael DeBakey and Scientific Director is Dr. A. M. Gotto. The aim of the Center is to launch a multidisciplinary attack on heart and blood vessel diseases. The Diet Modification Program is an attempt to demonstrate the effectiveness of *community* diet education programs for lowering plasma cholesterol and triglyceride levels. The target population includes the general public contacted through the mass media and certain preselected groups. We are attempting to establish a model which will be replicable for use in other communities.

The program uses both nutritional and behavioral information. We call the basic nutritional information we use in the program the HELP Your Heart Eating Plan (Gotto, Scott, Foreyt, and Reeves, 1975). This plan is designed to lower blood cholesterol and triglyceride levels. It recommends that participants achieve and maintain ideal body weight, eat less saturated fat, more poly-unsaturated fat, and reduce their intake of foods high in cholesterol (see Chapter 8).

Individuals responding to information they saw and heard in the mass media were invited to participate in the program. The initial study population during Year 1 consists of 250 individuals who expressed interest in participating. They were randomized into one of three groups:

Group A: This group consists of individuals participating at a minimal level. They receive a copy of the project's HELP Your Heart Eating Plan Booklet and are asked to report to our clinic for a blood test and other measures (weight, blood pressure, triceps skin fold, and questionnaire data) at their initial visit and at 3, 6, 12, 24, and 36 months.

Group B: In addition to receiving the project's HELP Your Heart Eating Plan Booklet, these participants receive additional nutritional information from a dietitian. Participants meet in groups of 8 to 10 for eight weekly sessions, then one session per month for the rest of the year (a total of 17 sessions over 12 months). Sessions last about 50 minutes. A blood test and other measures are taken at their initial visit and at 3, 6, 12, 24, and 36 months. Each meeting contains a specific nutrition lesson. Eight slide/tape presentations are shown, one each week, and discussed. These 8-minute slide/tape shows, developed by our staff, include:

1. Cardiovascular Disease
2. Fats and Cholesterol
3. Meat, Fish, and Poultry
4. Dairy Products
5. Food Selection
6. Foods Away from Home
7. Weight Loss
8. Special Foods

Group C: In addition to receiving the project's HELP Your Heart Eating Plan, participants receive the same nutritional information as the participants in Group B. They also receive training in a number of behavioral techniques from a dietitian. They meet in groups of 8 to 10 for eight weekly sessions, then one session per month for the rest of the year (a total of 17 sessions over 12 months). Sessions last 50 minutes. A blood test and other measurements are taken at their initial visit and at 3, 6, 12, 24, and 36 months. Each meeting includes a nutrition lesson and a specific behavior modification lesson. These behavior modification lessons include instruction in both the self-managed antecedent stimulus control techniques (self-monitored goal setting, self-initiated environmental planning) and the self-initiated consequent control techniques (self-reinforcement, self-punishment, and self-initiated environmental reinforcement).

The difference in Group C from Group B is the addition of these behavioral techniques. Group C participants are taught how to restructure their environment to increase the likelihood that they will modify their eating habits in accordance with the principles of the HELP Your Heart Eating Plan. Specifically, they receive behavioral training in each phase of dietary behavior:

1. Buying food
2. Storing food
3. Preparing food
4. Serving food
5. Eating food
6. Cleaning up food
7. Eating out

One of the principles of the HELP Your Heart Plan is to reduce to ideal body weight. Although weight reduction is not a major goal in our program, those participants needing to lose weight can do so by following the information they receive in the above training lessons and by following additional techniques that are made available to them:

1. Contingency contracting
2. Response blockage
3. Distributed eating
4. Relaxation training

The two major dependent variables in our study are plasma cholesterol and triglycerides. If the HELP Your Heart Eating

Plan is followed, participants will reduce both cholesterol and tri-glycerides by 10 percent. The Framingham study suggests that a 10 percent reduction in the serum cholesterol levels of the population would yield a 23 percent decrease in the incidence of heart disease (Cornfield, 1970). If patients maintain their change in eating habits and continue to follow the nutritional and behavioral information they learned as participants, cholesterol and trigly-cerides will continue to be lowered during the three-year follow-up period. A total of 1000 individuals are expected to participate in this phase of the program over the next three years. Preliminary data are encouraging and will be reported when complete.

Other dependent variables that we are looking at include blood pressure, weight, and triceps skin fold. All participants take a project questionnaire at various intervals which attempts to meas-ure eating patterns. We hope that as blood lipids change, change will also be reported in the kinds of foods eaten by the participants.

We have two other phases in our study, in addition to this program developed for the general public. Working closely with the Texas Agricultural Extension Service of the Texas A & M University system, we have developed a program for their Home Demonstration Clubs (HDC). The Home Demonstration Clubs have been a part of the Extension Service since the 1920's. These clubs are organized groups that conduct monthly programs for their members on topics in home economics. The clubs are nation-wide. In Texas alone, there are 1,462 clubs with over 24,000 mem-bers in 210 counties. In the Houston area, there are 16 active clubs and we are working with all of them. We have developed a program of nutrition education designed especially for the HDC members, and we are presently working with over 300 partici-pants in this program. The same measures are taken at the initial visit and at 3, 6, 12, 24, and 36 months.

The third phase of our study will begin later this year. Again working closely with the Texas Agricultural Extension Service of Texas A & M University System, we are designing a program to meet the needs of their Expanded Nutrition Program (ENP), a nationwide program initiated in 1969 to help low-income inner city families acquire knowledge and skills necessary to achieve more adequate diets. In the ENP program, education is conducted by neighborhood aides through home visits. These neighborhood aides will be trained by our staff to teach the principles of the HELP Your Heart Eating Plan to the participants. We hope that we will be able to reach sizeable black and Mexican-American populations through the ENP program. A total of 1000 participants are expected to participate in HDC and ENP phases of the program over the next four years.

In conclusion, the ultimate hope of our program is that by lowering plasma cholesterol and triglyceride concentrations through nutritional and behavioral information, these changes will lead to a slowing in the progression and severity of coronary heart disease and a decrease in the incidence of heart attacks. If successful, the model may be a useful one for attacking other risk factors such as hypertension and lack of exercise. We hope that the combination of nutrition and behavior modification techniques will indeed make a significant contribution to combating the number one killer in our society, heart disease.

References

Abrahms, J. L., and Allen, G. J. Comparative effectiveness of situational programming, financial pay-offs and group pressure in weight reduction. *Behavior Therapy*, 1974, *5*, 391-400.

Abramson, E. E. The effects of neurotic anxiety and objective fear on the eating behavior of obese and normal weight individuals. *Dissertation Abstracts International*, 1971, *32*, 1201.

Abramson, E. E. A review of behavioral approaches to weight control. *Behaviour Research and Therapy*, 1973, *11*, 547-556.

Air Force Diet. Toronto, Canada: Air Force Diet Publishers, 1960.

American Dental Association. School diet and dental health, resolution reaffirmed by the Board of Trustees, 1961.

American Dietetic Association and American Diabetes Association. *Meal planning with exchange lists. Revised.* New York: American Dietetic Association and American Diabetes Association, 1956.

American Heart Association. *The way to a man's heart.* New York: American Heart Association, 1972.

American Heart Association. *1974 Heart Facts.* New York: American Heart Association, 1974.

American Medical Association Council on Foods and Nutrition. Review of Dr. Atkins' diet revolution. Unpublished manuscript, 1973.

Arthur, A. Z. Diagnostic testing and the new alternatives. *Psychological Bulletin*, 1969, *72*, 183-192.

Atkins, R. C. *Dr. Atkins' diet revolution: The high calorie way to stay thin forever.* New York: David McKay Company, Inc., 1972.

Ayllon, T. Intensive treatment of psychotic behavior by stimulus satiation and food reinforcement. *Behaviour Research and Therapy*, 1963, *1*, 53-61.

Bandura, A. *Principles of behavior modification.* New York: Holt, Rinehart and Winston, 1969.

Bennett, I., and Simon, M. *The prudent diet.* New York: David White, 1973.

Bergin, A. E. The evaluation of therapeutic outcomes. In A. E. Bergin and S. L. Garfield (Eds.), *Handbook of psychotherapy and behavior change: An empirical analysis.* New York: Wiley, 1971, pp. 217-270.

Bergin, A. E., and Garfield, S. L. (Eds.) *Handbook of psychotherapy and behavior change: An empirical analysis.* New York: Wiley, 1971.

197

Bernard, J. L. Rapid treatment of gross obesity by operant techniques. *Psychological Reports*, 1968, *23*, 663-666.

Bloom, W. L., and Azar, G. J. Similarities of carbohydrate deficiency and fasting: Weight loss, electrolyte excretion, and fatigue. *Archives of Internal Medicine*, 1963, *112*, 333-343.

Bookbinder, L. J. Simple conditioning vs. the dynamic approach to symptoms and symptom substitution: A reply to Yates. *Psychological Reports*, 1962, *10*, 71-77.

Bradfield, R. B., Paulos, J., and Grossman, M. A. Energy expenditure and heart rate of obese high school girls. *American Journal of Clinical Nutrition*, 1971, *24*, 1482-1488.

Bray, G. A. The myth of diet in the management of obesity. *American Journal of Clinical Nutrition*, 1970, *23*, 1141-1148.

Breger, L., and McGaugh, J. Critique and reformulation of 'learning theory' approaches to psychotherapy and neurosis. *Psychological Bulletin*, 1965, *63*, 338-358.

Bruch, H. Psychiatric aspects of obesity in children. *American Journal of Psychiatry*, 1943, *99*, 752-761.

Bruch, H. *Eating disorders: Obesity, anorexia nervosa, and the person within.* New York: Basic Books, Inc., 1973.

Brunzell, J. D., Hazzard, W. R., Porte, D. Jr., and Bierman, E. L. Evidence for a common, saturable, triglyceride removal mechanism for chylomicrons and very low density lipoproteins in man. *Journal of Clinical Investigation*, 1973, *52*, 1578-1585.

Bullen, B. A., Reed, R. B., and Mayer, J. Physical activity of obese and non-obese adolescent girls appraised by motion picture sampling. *American Journal of Clinical Nutrition*, 1964, *14*, 211-223.

Burkett, D. Some disease characteristics of modern western civilization. *British Medical Journal*, 1973, *3*, 224-228.

Cabanac, M. Physiological role of pleasure. *Science*, 1971, *173*, 1103-1107.

Cabanac, M., and Ducleaux, R. Obesity: Absence of satiety aversion to sucrose. *Science*, 1970, *168*, 496-497.

Cabanac, M., Ducleaux, R., and Spector, N. Sensory feedback in regulation of body weight: Is there a ponderostat? *Nature*, 1971, *229*, 125-127.

Cahill, G. F., Jr. Physiology of insulin in man. *Diabetes*, 1971, *20*, 785-799.

Cahoon, D. D. Symptom substitution and the behavior therapies. *Psychological Bulletin*, 1968, *69*, 149-157.

Campbell, R. G., Hashim, S. A., and Van Itallie, T. B. Responses to variation in nutritive density in lean and obese subjects. *New England Journal of Medicine*, 1971, *285*, 1402-1407.

Cautela, J. R. Treatment of compulsive behavoir by covert sensitization. *Psychological Record*, 1966, *16*, 33-41.

Cautela, J. R. Covert sensitization. *Psychological Reports*, 1967, *20*, 459-468.

Chapman, J. M., and Massey, F. J. Jr. The interrelationship of serum cholesterol, hypertension, body weight, and risk of coronary disease. Results of the first ten years' follow-up in the Los Angeles heart study. *Journal of Chronic Diseases*, 1964, 17, 933-949.

Choate, R. B. Testimony before the House Select Committee on Small Business, June 11, 1971.

Christakis, G., Rinzler, S. H., Archer, M., Winslow, G., Jampel, S., Stephenson, J., Friedman, G., Fein, H., Kraus, A., and James, G. A dietary approach to the prevention of coronary heart disease—a seven year report. *American Journal of Public Health*, 1966, *56*, 299-314.

Christensen, E. R., Jeffrey, D. B., and Pappas, J. P. *A therapist manual for a behavior modification weight reduction program.* Research and development report No. 37, Counseling and Psychological Services, University of Utah, 1973.

Computer Diet. *Ladies' Home Journal*, January, 1965, *82*, 62-65.

Conrad, E. H. Psychogenic obesity: The effects of social rejection upon hunger, food-craving and food-consumption and the drive-reduction value of eating for obese vs. normal individuals. *Dissertation Abstracts International*, 1970, *30*, 4787-4788.

Cornfield, J. Design of primary and secondary prevention trials. *Atherosclerosis Proceedings of the Second International Symposium*. New York: Springer-Verlag, Inc., 1970, pp. 566-571.

Cronbach, J., and Furby, L. How we should measure "change"—or should we? *Psychological Bulletin*, 1970, *74*, 68-80.

Crowne, D. P., and Marlowe, D. *The approval motive*. New York: Wiley, 1964.

Dallas Independent School District, *Administration Code 2480.5*. Dallas, Texas, 1975.

Davidson, P. O., Clark, F. W., and Hamerlynck, L. A. *Evaluation of behavioral programs*. Champaign, Ill.: Research Press, 1974.

Davison, G. C., Tsujimoto, R. N., and Glaros, A. G. Attribution and the maintenance of behavior change of falling asleep. *Journal of Abnormal Psychology*, 1973, *82*, 124-133.

Davison, G. C., and Valins, S. Maintenance of self-attributed and drug-attributed behavior change. *Journal of Personality and Social Psychology*, 1969, *11*, 25-33.

Dawber, T. R., Kannel, W. B., and McNamara, P. M. The prediction of coronary heart disease. *Transactions of the Association of Life Insurance Medical Directors of America*, 1964, *47*, 70-105.

Dawber, T. R., Kannel, W. B., Revotskie, N., and Kagan, A. The epidemiology of coronary heart diseases. The Framingham inquiry. *Proceedings of the Royal Society of Medicine*, 1962, *55*, 265-271.

Decke, E. Effects of taste on the eating behavior of obese and normal persons. Cited in S. Schacter, *Emotion, obesity, and crime*. New York: Academic Press, 1971.

Dorris, R. J., and Stunkard, A. J. Physical activity: Performance and attitudes of a group of obese women. *American Journal of Medical Sciences*, 1957, *233*, 622-628.

Drew Chemical Corporation. *Fats and oils: Fatty acid composition and physical properties*. Parsippany, New Jersey: Drew Chemical Corporation, undated.

Dukes, W. F. N = 1. *Psychological Bulletin*, 1965, *64*, 74-79.

D'Zurilla, T. J., and Goldfried, M. R. Problem solving and behavior modification. *Journal of Abnormal Psychology*, 1971, *78*, 107-126.

Elashoff, J. D. Analysis of covariance: A delicate instrument. *American Educational Research Journal*, 1969, *6*, 383-402.

Eysenck, H. J. Learning theory and behavior therapy. *Journal of Mental Science*, 1959, *105*, 61-75.

Eysenck, H. J. Editorial. *Behaviour Research and Therapy*, 1963, *1*, 1-2.

Eysenck, H. J. Behavior therapy and its critics. *Journal of Behavior Therapy and Experimental Psychiatry*, 1970, *1*, 5-15.

Eysenck, H. J. Behavior therapy as a scientific discipline. *Journal of Consulting and Clinical Psychology*, 1971, *36*, 314-319.

Eysenck, S., and Eysenck, H. An improved short questionnaire for the measurement of extraversion and neuroticism. *Life Sciences*, 1964, *3*, 1103-1109.

Eysenck, H. J., and Rachman, S. *The causes and cures of neurosis.* San Diego, Calif.: Robert R. Knapp, 1965.

Fee, J. M., Wilson, N. L., and Wilson, R. H. L. Obesity: A gross national product. In N. L. Wilson (Ed.), *Obesity.* Philadelphia: F. A. Davis, 1969, pp. 238-245.

Feeley, R. M., Criner, P. E., and Watt, B. K. Cholesterol content of foods. *Journal of the American Dietetic Association*, 1972, *61*, 134-149.

Feinstein, A. R. The measurement of success in weight reduction: An analysis of methods and a new index. *Journal of Chronic Diseases*, 1959, *10*, 439-456.

Feinstein, A. R. How do we measure accomplishment in weight reduction? In L. Lasagna (Ed.), *Obesity: Causes, consequences, and treatment.* New York: Med Com Press, 1974, pp. 81-87.

Feldman, M. P., and MacCulloch, M. D. *Homosexual behaviour: Therapy and assessment.* Oxford: Pergamon Press, 1971.

Feldt, L. S. A comparison of the precision of three experimental designs employing a concomitant variable. *Psychometrika*, 1958, *23*, 335-353.

Ferster, C. B., Nurnberger, J. I., and Levitt, E. B. The control of eating. *Journal of Mathetics*, 1962, *1*, 87-109.

Ferster, C. B., and Perrott, M. C. *Behavior principles.* New York: Meredith Corporation, 1968.

Fiske, D. W., Hunt, H. F., Luborsky, L., Orne, M. T., Parloff, M. B., Reiser, M. F., and Tuma, A. H. Planning of research on effectiveness of psychotherapy. *Archives of General Psychiatry*, 1970, *22*, 22-32.

Foreyt, J. P. (Ed.) *Behavioral treatments of obesity.* New York: Pergamon Press, in press.

Foreyt, J. P., and Kennedy, W. A. Treatment of overweight by aversion therapy. *Behaviour Research and Therapy*, 1971, *9*, 29-34.

Fowler, R. S. Jr., Fordyce, W. E., Boyd, V. D., and Masock, A. J. The mouthful diet: A behavioral approach to overeating. *Rehabilitation Psychology*, 1972, *19*, 98-106.

Fredrickson, D. S., and Levy, R. I. Fimilial hyperlipoproteinemia. In J. B. Stanbury, J. B. Wyngaarden, and D. S. Fredrickson (Eds.), *The metabolic basis of inherited disease.* New York: McGraw-Hill, 1972, pp. 545-614.

Fredrickson, D. S., Levy, R. I., and Lees, R. S. Fat transport in lipoproteins—an integrated approach to mechanisms and disorders. *New England Journal of Medicine*, 1967, *267*, 36-44, 94-103, 148-156, 215-225, 273-281.

Frohwirth, R. A. Aversive conditioning treatment of overweight. Unpublished doctoral dissertation, The Florida State University, 1974.

Fujita, Y., Gotto, A. M., Jr., and Unger, R. H. Basal and post-protein insulin and glucagon levels during a high and low carbohydrate intake and their relationships to plasma triglycerides. *Diabetes*, 1975, in press.

Gaul, D. J., Craighead, W. E., and Mahoney, M. J. The relationship between eating rates and obesity. *Journal of Consulting and Clinical Psychology*, 1975, *43*, 123-125.

Gilbert, D. G. Taste in underweight, overweight, and normal-weight subjects before and after sucrose ingestion. Unpublished master's thesis, Florida State University, 1973.

Glick, G. Effect of physical activity on body weight and body fat of obese, normal weight and underweight young males. *Israel Journal of Medical Science*, 1974, *10*, 289.

Goldman, R., Jaffa, M., and Schachter, S. Yom Kippur, Air France, dormitory food, and the eating behavior of obese and normal persons. *Journal of Personality and Social Psychology*, 1968, *10*, 117-123.

Goldstein, J. L., Dana, S. E., Brunschede, G. Y., and Brown, M. S. Genetic heterogeneity in familial hypercholesterolemia: Evidence for two different mutations affecting functions of low-density lipoprotein receptor. *Proceedings of the National Academy of Sciences*, 1975, *72*, 1092-1096.

Goldstein, J. L., Hazzard, W. R., Schrott, H. G., Bierman, E. L., and Motulsky, A. G. Hyperlipidemia in coronary heart disease. I. Lipid levels in 500 survivors of myocardial infarction. *Journal of Clinical Investigation*, 1973, *52*, 1533-1542.

Goldstein, J. L., Schrott, H. G., Hazzard, W. R., Bierman, E. L., and Motulsky, A. G. Hyperlipidemia in coronary heart disease. II. Genetic analysis of lipid levels in 176 families and delineation of a new inherited disorder, combined hyperlipidemia. *Journal of Clinical Investigation*, 1973, *52*, 1544-1568.

Gotto, A. M., Jr., Scott, L. W., Foreyt, J. P., and Reeves, R. *HELP Your Heart Eating Plan.* (Booklet). Houston, Texas: Baylor College of Medicine, 1975.

Grande, F., Anderson, J. T., Taylor, H. L., and Keys, A. Basal metabolic rate in man in semi-starvation and refeeding. *Federation Proceedings*, 1957, *16*, 49-50. (Abstract)

Grinker, J. Behavioral and metabolic consequences of weight reduction. *Journal of the American Dietetic Association*, 1973, *62*, 30-34.

Grinker, J., and Hirsch, J. Metabolic and behavioral correlates of obesity. In CIBA Foundation Symposium 8 (new series), *Physiology, emotion and psychosomatic illness.* Amsterdam: Associated Scientific, 1972, 349-374.

Gussow, J. Counternutritional messages of TV ads aimed at children. *Journal of Nutrition Education*, 1972, *4*, 48-52.

Hagen, R. L. Group therapy versus bibliotherapy in weight reduction. *Behavior Therapy*, 1974, *5*, 222-234.

Hagen, R. L., Foreyt, J., and Durham, T. The drop out problem: Reducing attrition in obesity research. *Behavior Therapy*, 1975, in press.

Hagen, R. L., Wollersheim, J., and Paul, G. Weight reduction manual. Unpublished manuscript, University of Illinois, 1969.

Hall, S. M. Self-control and therapist control in the behavioral treatment of overweight women. *Behaviour Research and Therapy*, 1972, *10*, 59-68.

Hall, S. M., and Hall, R. G. Outcome and methodological consideration in behavioral treatment of obesity. *Behavior Therapy*, 1974, *5*, 352-364.

Hall, S. M., Hall, R. G., Hanson, R. W., and Borden, B. L. Permanence of two self-managed treatments of overweight in university and community populations. *Journal of Consulting and Clinical Psychology*, 1974, *42*, 781-786.

Harmatz, M. G., and Lapuc, P. Behavior modification of overeating in a psychiatric population. *Journal of Consulting and Clinical Psychology*, 1968, *32*, 583-587.

Harris, C. W. *Problems in measuring change.* Madison: University of Wisconsin Press, 1963.

Harris, M. B. Self-directed program for weight control: A pilot study. *Journal of Abnormal Psychology*, 1969, *74*, 263-270.

Harris, M. B., and Bruner, C. G. A comparison of a self-control and a contract procedure for weight control. *Behaviour Research and Therapy*, 1971, *9*, 347-354.

Harris, M. B., and Hallbauer, E. S. Self-directed weight control through eating and exercise. *Behaviour Research and Therapy*, 1973, *11*, 523-529.

Harvey, W. *On corpulence in relation to disease.* London: Henry Renshaw, 1872.

Hashim, S. A., and Van Itallie, T. B. Studies in normal and obese subjects with a monitored food dispensary device. *Annals of the New York Academy of Science*, 1965, *131*, 654-661.

Heuston, H. Fitness at Phillips Petroleum. *Fitness for Living*, 1973, May-June, 74-79.

Hirsch, J. Adipose cellularity in relation to human obesity. *Advances in Internal Medicine*, 1971, *17*, 289-300.

Hirsch, J. Can we modify the number of adipose cells? *Postgraduate Medicine*, 1972, *51*, 83-86.

Hirsch, J., and Han, P. W. Cellularity of rat adipose tissue: Effects of growth, starvation, and obesity. *Journal of Lipid Research*, 1969, *10*, 77-82.

Hirsch, J., Knittle, J. L., and Salans, L. B. Cell lipid content and cell number in obese and nonobese human adipose tissue. *Journal of Clinical Investigation*, 1966, *45*, 1023.

Hollingshead, A. B., and Redlich, F. C. *Social class and mental illness.* New York: Wiley, 1958.

Horan, J. J., and Johnson, R. G. Coverant conditioning through a self-management application of the Premack principle: Its effect on weight reduction. *Journal of Behavior Therapy and Experimental Psychiatry*, 1971, *2*, 243-249.

Huenemann, R. L. Environmental factors associated with preschool obesity (II). *Journal of the American Dietetic Association*, 1974, *64*, 480-487.

Innes, J. A., Campbell, I. W., Campbell, C. J., Needle, A. L., and Munro, J. F. Long-term follow-up of therapeutic starvation. *British Medical Journal*, 1974, *2*, 356-359.

Inter-Society Commission for Heart Disease Resources, Atherosclerosis and Epidemiology Study Groups. Primary Prevention of the Atherosclerotic Disease. *Circulation*, 1970, *42*, 55-95.

Jackson, D. Interference proneness and sensitivity to meal palatability in the obese and nonobese. Unpublished master's thesis, University of Cincinnati, 1973.

Jacobs, J. *The death and life of great American cities.* New York: Vintage Books, 1961.

Jameson, G., and Williams, E. *The drinking man's diet.* San Francisco: Cameron and Co., 1964.

Janda, L. H., and Rimm, D. C. Covert sensitization in the treatment of obesity. *Journal of Abnormal Psychology*, 1972, *80*, 37-42.

Jeffrey, D. B. A comparison of the effects of external control and self-control on the modification and maintenance of weight. *Journal of Abnormal Psychology*, 1974, *83*, 404-410. (b)

Jeffrey, D. B. Some methodological issues in research on obesity. *Psychological Reports*, 1974, *35*, 623-626. (a)

Jeffrey, D. B. The potential side effects in external control and self-control contingency systems for weight loss. Paper presented at the Eighth Annual Convention of the Association for the Advancement of Behavior Therapy, Chicago, Illinois, November, 1974.

Jeffrey, D. B. Treatment evaluation issues in research on addictive behaviors. *Addictive Behaviors*, 1975, 1, 23-36.

Jeffrey, D. B. Behavioral management of obesity. In W. E. Craighead, A. E. Kazdin, and M. J. Mahoney (Eds.), *Behavior modification: Principles, issues, and applications*. New York: Houghton, Mifflin, in press. (a)

Jeffrey, D. B. Additional methodological considerations in the behavioral treatment of obesity: A reply to the Hall and Hall review of obesity. *Behavior Therapy*, 1975, 6, 96-97.

Jeffrey, D. B. Self-control approaches to the management of obesity. In J. P. Foreyt (Ed.), *Behavioral Treatments of Obesity*. New York: Pergamon Press, in press. (b)

Jeffrey, D. B., and Christensen, E. R. The relative efficacy of behavior therapy, will power, and no-treatment control procedures for weight loss. Paper presented at the meeting of the Association for the Advancement of Behavior Therapy, New York, October, 1972.

Jeffrey, D. B., and Christensen, E. R. Behavior therapy versus "will power" in the management of obesity. *The Journal of Psychology*, 1975, 90, 303-311.

Jecrey, D. B., and Katz, R. C. *A Behavioral Self-Control Approach to Dietary, Exercise, and Psychological Management*. Englewood Cliffs, N. J.: Prentice-Hall, in press.

Jeffrey, D. B., Christensen, E. R., and Katz, R. C. Behavior therapy weight reduction programs: Some preliminary findings on the need for follow-up. *Psychotherapy: Theory, Research and Practice*, in press.

Jeffrey, D. B., Christensen, E. R., and Pappas, J. P. A case study report of a behavioral modification weight reduction group: Treatment and follow-up. *Research and Development Report* No. 33, University of Utah Counseling Center, 1972.

Jeffrey, D. D., Christensen, E. R., and Pappas, J. P. Developing a behavioral program and therapist manual for the treatment of obesity. *Journal of the American Health Association*, 1973, 21, 455-459.

Johnson, M. L., Burke, B. S., and Mayer, J. Relative importance of inactivity and overeating in the energy balance of obese high school girls. *American Journal of Clinical Nutrition*, 1956, 4, 37.

Jordan, H. A. In defense of body weight. *Journal of the American Dietetic Association*, 1973, 62, 17-21. (a)

Jordan, H. A. Physiological control of food intake in man. Paper presented at the Fogarty International Conference on Obesity, Washington, D. C., October 1-3, 1973. (b)

Jordan, H. A., and Levitz, L. S. A behavioral approach to the problem of obesity. *Obesity and Bariatric Medicine*, 1975, 4, 58-69.

Kanfer, F. H., and Phillips, J. S. *Learning foundations of behavior therapy*. New York: John Wiley & Sons, 1970.

Kannel, W. B., Castelli, W. P., Gordon, T., and McNamara, P. M. Serum cholesterol, lipoproteins, and the risk of coronary heart disease. The Framingham study. *Annals of Internal Medicine*, 1971, 74, 1-12.

Karp, S. A., and Pardes, H. Psychological differentiation (field dependence) in obese women. *Psychosomatic Medicine*, 1965, 27, 238-244.

Keller, F. S. Neglected rewards in the educational process. Paper read at the 23rd Annual Meeting of the American Conference of Academic Deans, Los Angeles, Calif., January 16, 1967.

Kennedy, B. J. Nutritionists apply self-control training, food exchange plan treatment, and no-treatment in the treatment of obesity. Unpublished master's thesis, University of Missouri, Columbia, 1972.

Kennedy, W. A., and Foreyt, J. P. Control of eating behavior in an obese patient by avoidance conditioning. *Psychological Reports*, 1968, *22*, 571-576.

Keys, A., Anderson, J. T., and Grande, F. Serum cholesterol response to changes in the diet. I. Iodine value of dietary fat versus 2S-P. *Metabolism*, 1965, *14*, 747-758.

Krasner, L. Behavior therapy. In P. H. Mussen and M. R. Rosenzweig (Eds.), *Annual Review of Psychology Vol. 22*. Palo Alto, California: Annual Reviews, Inc., 1971.

Lazarus, A. A., and Davison, G. C. Clinical innovation in research and practice. In A. E. Bergin and S. L. Garfield (Eds.), *Handbook of psychotherapy and behavior change: An empirical analysis*. New York: John Wiley & Sons, 1971.

Leon, G. R., and Chamberlain, K. Emotional arousal, eating patterns, and body image as differential factors associated with varying success in maintaining a weight loss. *Journal of Consulting and Clinical Psychology*, 1973, *40*, 474-480.

Lincoln, J. E. Calorie intake, obesity, and physical activity. *American Journal of Clinical Nutrition*, 1972, *25*, 390-394.

Linton, P. H., Conley, M., Kuechenmeister, C., and McClusky, H. Satiety and obesity. *American Journal of Clinical Nutrition*, 1972, *25*, 368-370.

Locke, E. A. Is "behavior therapy" behavioristic: An analysis of Wolpe's psychotherapeutic methods. *Psychological Bulletin*, 1971, *76*, 318-327.

London, A. M., and Schreiber, E. D. A controlled study of the effects of group discussions and an anorexiant in outpatient treatment of obesity with attention to the psychological aspects of dieting. *Annals of Internal Medicine*, 1966, *65*, 80-92.

London, P. The end of ideology in behavior modification. *American Psychologist*, 1972, *27*, 913-926.

Mahoney, M. J. Self-control strategies in weight loss. Paper presented at the meeting of the Association for the Advancement of Behavior Therapy, New York, October, 1972.

Mahoney, M. J. *Cognition and behavior modification*. Cambridge, Mass.: Ballinger, 1974. (b)

Mahoney, M. J. Self-reward and self-monitoring techniques for weight control. *Behavior Therapy*, 1974, *5*, 48-57. (a)

Mahoney, M. J. Fat fiction. *Behavior Therapy*, 1975, *6*, 416-418 (a).

Mahoney, M. J. The obese eating style: Bites, beliefs, and behavior modification. *Addictive Behaviors*, 1975, in press. (b)

Mahoney, M. J. and Jeffrey, D. B. A manual of self-control procedures for the overweight. Abstracted in the JSAS *Catalog of Selected Documents in Psychology*, 1974, *4*, 129.

Mahoney, K., and Mahoney, M. J. Cognitive factors in weight reduction. In J. D. Krumboltz and C. E. Thoresen (Eds.), *Counseling methods*. New York: Holt, Rinehart & Winston, 1975.

Mahoney, M. J., and Mahoney, K. *Weight control as a personal science*. New York: W. W. Norton, in press.

Mahoney, M. J., Moura, N. G. M., and Wade, T. C. The relative efficacy of self-reward, self-punishment, and self-monitoring techniques for weight loss. *Journal of Consulting and Clinical Psychology*, 1973, *40*, 404-407.

Mann, R. A. The behavior-therapeutic use of contingency contracting to control an adult behavior problem: Weight control. *Journal of Applied Behavior Analysis*, 1972, *5*, 99-109.

Manno, B., and Marston, A. R. Weight reduction as a function of negative covert reinforcement (sensitization) versus positive covert reinforcement. *Behaviour Research and Therapy*, 1972, *10*, 201-207.

Martin, J. E., and Sachs, D. A. The effects of a self-control weight loss program on an obese woman. *Journal of Behavior Therapy and Experimental Psychiatry*, 1973, *4*, 155-159.

Martin, S. A course in behavior modification. University of Houston, Houston, Texas, Department of Psychology, 1973.

Maxfield, E., and Konishi, F. Patterns of food intake and physical activity in obesity. *Journal of the American Dietetic Association*, 1966, *49*, 406-408.

Mayer, J. *Overweight: Causes, cost, and control.* Englewood Cliffs, N. J.: Prentice Hall, 1968.

Mayer, J., Marshall, N. B., Vitale, J. J., Christensen, S. H., Mashayekhi, M. B., and Stare, F. J. Exercise, food intake, and body weight in normal rats and genetically obese adult mice. *American Journal of Physiology*, 1954, *177*, 544-548.

Mayer, J., and Thomas, D. W. Regulation of food intake and obesity. *Science*, 1967, *156*, 328-337.

McCarthy, M. C. Dietary and activity patterns of obese women in Trinidad. *Journal of the American Dietetic Association*, 1966, *48*, 33-37.

McKenna, R. J. Some effects of anxiety level and food cues on the eating behavior of obese and normal subjects: A comparison of the Schachterian and psychosomatic conceptions. *Journal of Personality and Social Psychology*, 1972, *22*, 320-325.

McReynolds, W., Lutz, R., Paulsen, B., and Kohrs, M. The effectiveness of two behavioral approaches to weight loss with nutritionists as therapists. Paper presented at the Eighth Annual Convention of the Association for the Advancement of Behavior Therapy, Chicago, Illinois, November, 1974.

Metropolitan Life Insurance Company. *You and your health.* New York: Metropolitan Life Insurance Company, 1973.

Metropolitan Life Insurance Company. New weight standards for men and women. *Statistical Bulletin*, 1959, *40*, (Whole No. 3).

Meyer, V., and Crisp, A. H. Aversion therapy in two cases of obesity. *Behaviour Research and Therapy*, 1964, *2*, 143-147.

Miettinen, M., Turpeinen, O., Karvonen, M. J., and Elosuo, R. Effects of cholesterol-lowering diet on mortality from coronary heart disease and other causes: A twelve year clinical trial in men and women. *Lancet*, 1972, *2*, 835-838.

Miettinen, T. A. Current views on cholesterol metabolism. In H. Greten, R. Levine, E. F. Pfeiffer, and A. E. Renold (Eds.), *Lipid metabolism, obesity, and diabetes mellitus: impact upon atherosclerosis. International symposium, April, 1972.* Stuttgart: Georg Thieme Publishers, 1974. Pp. 37-44.

Miller, C. New perspectives on obesity. Paper presented at Florida Psychological Association, Miami, Florida, May, 1974.

Moore, C. H., and Crum, B. C. Weight reduction in a chronic schizophrenic by means of operant conditioning procedures: A case study. *Behaviour Research and Therapy*, 1969, *7*, 129-131.

Musante, G. J. The Dietary Rehabilitation Clinic: Evaluative report of a behavioral and dietary treatment of obesity. *Behavior Therapy*, in press.

National Academy of Sciences. *Recommended Dietary Allowances, 8th edition.* Washington, D. C.: Food and Nutrition Board of the National Academy of Sciences National Research Council, 1974.

National Center for Health Statistics. *1974 Heart Facts Reference Sheet.* New York: American Heart Association, 1974.

Nisbett, R. E. Determinants of food intake in human obesity. *Science*, 1968, *159*, 1254-1255. (a)

Nisbett, R. E. Taste, deprivation, and weight determinants of eating behavior. *Journal of Personality and Social Psychology*, 1968, *10*, 107-116. (b)

Nisbett, R. E. Hunger, obesity, and the ventromedial hypothalamus. *Psychological Review*, 1972, *79*, 433-453.

Nisbett, R. E., Hanson, L. R. Jr., Harris, A., and Stair, A. Taste responsiveness, weight loss, and the ponderostat. *Physiology and Behavior*, 1973, *11*, 641-645.

Patterson, G. R. A community mental health program for children. In L. A. Hamerlynck, P. O. Davidson, and L. Acher (Eds.), *Behavior modification and the ideal mental health services.* Calgary: University of Calgary, 1969, pp. 131-179.

Patterson, G. R., Ray, R. S., and Shaw, D. R. Direct intervention in families of deviant children. *Oregon Research Institute Research Bulletin*, 1968, *8*, No. 9.

Paul, G. L. Behavior modification research: Design and tactics. In C. M. Franks (Ed.), *Behavior therapy: Appraisal and status.* New York: McGraw-Hill, 1969, pp. 29-62.

Paulsen, B., McReynolds, W. T., Lutz, R. N., and Kohrs, M. B. Effective weight control through behavior modification and nutrition education: A treatment manual. Unpublished paper, Lincoln University, 1974.

Penick, S. B., Filion, R., Fox, S., and Stunkard, A. J. Behavior modification in the treatment of obesity. *Psychosomatic Medicine*, 1971, *33*, 49-55.

Penick, S. B., and Stunkard, A. J. The treatment of obesity. *Advances in Psychosomatic Medicine*, 1972, 7, 217-228.

Pennington, Q. W. Treatment of obesity with calorically unrestricted diets. *American Journal of Clinical Nutrition*, 1953, *1*, 343-348.

Pliner, P. L. Effects of cue salience on the behavior of obese and normal subjects. *Journal of Abnormal Psychology*, 1973, *82*, 226-232.

Pliner, P., Meyer, P., and Blankstein, K. Responsiveness to affective stimuli by obese and normal individuals. *Journal of Abnormal Psychology*, 1974, *83*, 74-80.

Pollock, M., Laughridge, E., Coleman, B., Linnerud, A., and Jackson, A. Prediction of body density in young and middle-aged women. *Journal of Applied Physiology* (in press).

Portes, A. On the emergence of behavior therapy in modern society. *Journal of Consulting and Clinical Psychology*, 1971, *36*, 303-313.

Price, J. M., and Grinker, J. Effects of degree of obesity, food deprivation, and palatability on eating behavior of humans. *Journal of Comparative and Physiological Psychology*, 1973, *85*, 265-271.

Rachman, S., and Eysenck, H. J. Reply to a "critique and reformulation" of behavior therapy. *Psychological Bulletin*, 1966, *65*, 167-169.

Rachman, S., and Teasdale, J. *Aversion therapy and behaviour disorders: An analysis.* Coral Gables, Florida: University of Miami Press, 1969.

Redgrave, T. G. Inhibition of protein synthesis and absorption of lipid into thoracic duct lymph in rats. *Proceedings for the Society of Experimental Biology and Medicine*, 1969, *130*, 776-780.

Risley, T. R. Behavior modification: An experimental-therapeutic endeavor. In L. A. Hamerlynck, P. O. Davidson, and L. Acker (Eds.), *Behavior modification and ideal mental health services.* Calgary: University of Calgary Press, 1969.

Rivlin, R. S. Drug Therapy: Therapy of obesity with hormones. *The New England Journal of Medicine, 1975, 292,* 26-29.

Rodin, J. Effects of distraction on performance of obese and normal subjects. *Journal of Comparative and Physiological Psychology, 1973, 88,* 68-75.

Rodin, J., Herman, C., and Schachter, S. Stimulus sensitivity in obese and normal persons. Unpublished paper, Columbia University, 1969.

Romanczyk, R. G., Tracey, D. A., Wilson, G. T., and Thorpe, G. L. Behavior techniques in the treatment of obesity: A comparative analysis. *Behaviour Research and Therapy, 1973, 11,* 629-640.

Rose, G. A., and Williams, R. T. Metabolic studies on large and small eaters. *British Journal of Nutrition, 1961, 15,* 1-9.

Ross, L. Cue and cognition-controlled eating among obese and normal subjects. *Dissertation Abstracts International,* 1970 (Dec.), *31* (6-B), 3693-4.

Rotter, J. Generalized expectancies for internal versus external control of reinforcement. *Psychological Monographs: General and Applied, 1966, 80,* 1-28.

Salans, L. B., Knittle, J. L., and Hirsch, J. The role of adipose cell enlargement in the carbohydrate intolerance of human obesity. *Journal of Clinical Investigation, 1967, 46,* 1112.

Salans, L. B., Knittle, J. L., and Hirsch, J. The role of adipose cell size and adipose tissue insulin sensitivity in the carbohydrate intolerance of human obesity. *Journal of Clinical Investigation, 1968, 47,* 153-165.

Schachter, S. Cognitive effects of bodily functioning: Studies of obesity and eating. In D. C. Glass (Ed.), *Biology and behavior: Neurophysiology and emotion.* New York: The Rockefeller University Press and Russell Sage Foundation, 1967, pp. 117-144.

Schachter, S. Obesity and eating. *Science, 1968, 161,* 751-756.

Schachter, S. *Emotion, obesity, and crime.* New York: Academic Press, 1971. (b)

Schachter, S. Some extraordinary facts about obese humans and rats. *American Psychologist, 1971, 26,* 129-144. (a)

Schachter, S., Goldman, R., and Gordon, A. Effects of fear, food deprivation, and obesity on eating. *Journal of Personality and Social Psychology, 1968, 10,* 91-97.

Schachter, S., and Gross, L. Manipulated time and eating behavior. *Journal of Personality and Social Psychology, 1968, 10,* 98-106.

Schachter, S., and Rodin, J. *Obese humans and rats.* Potomac, Md.: Lawrence Erlbaum, 1974.

Schiffman, S. S. The dietary rehabilitation clinic: A multi-aspect, dietary, and behavioral approach to the treatment of obesity. Paper presented at Association for Advancement of Behavior Therapy, Miami Beach, Florida, December, 1973.

Schwarz, K. Recent dietary trace element research, exemplified by tin, fluorine, and silicon. *Federation Proceedings, 1974, 33,* 1748-1757.

Sims, E. A. H., Bray, G. A., Danforth, E. Jr., Glennon, J. A., Horton, E. S., Salans, L. B., and O'Connell, M. Experimental obesity in man. VI: The effect of variations in intake of carbohydrate on carbohydrate, lipid, and cortisol metabolism. In H. Greten, R. Levine, E. F. Pfeiffer, and A. E. Renold (Eds.), *Lipid metabolism, obesity, diabetes mellitus: Impact upon atherosclerosis.*

International symposium, April, 1972. Stuttgart: Georg Thieme Publishers, 1974. Pp. 70-77.

Singh, D. Role of response habits and cognitive factors in determination of behavior of obese humans. *Journal of Personality and Social Psychology,* 1973, 27, 220-238.

Skinner, B. F. What is psychotic behavior? In T. Gildea (Ed.), *Theory and treatment of the psychoses.* Washington University Studies, 1956.

Skinner, B. F. What is the experimental analysis of behavior? *Journal of the Experimental Analysis of Behavior,* 1966, 9, 213-218.

Slack, J. Risks of ischaemic heart disease in familial hyperlipoproteinaemic states. *Lancet,* 1969, 2, 1380-1382.

Sobell, M. B., and Sobell, L. C. The need for realism, relevance and operational assumptions in the study of substance dependence. Paper presented at the International Symposia on Alcohol and Drug Research, Addiction Research Foundation, Toronto, Canada, October, 1973.

Stamler, J. Epidemiology of coronary heart disease. *Medical Clinics of North America,* 1973, 57, 5-46.

Stefanik, P. A., Heald, F. P. Jr., and Mayer, J. Caloric intake in relation to energy output of obese and non-obese adolescent boys. *American Journal of Clinical Nutrition,* 1959, 7, 55-62.

Stein, O., and Stein, Y. The removal of cholesterol from Landschütz ascites cells by high-density apolipoprotein. *Biochimica et Biophysica Acta,* 1973, 326, 232-244.

Stein, O., Stein, Y., Goodman, D. S., and Fidge, N. H. The metabolism of chylomicron cholesteryl ester in rat liver. *Journal of Cell Biology,* 1969, 43, 410-431.

Stillman, I. M., and Baker, S. S. *The doctor's quick weight loss diet.* Englewood Cliffs, N. J.: Prentice Hall, 1967.

Storms, M. D., and Nisbett, R. E. Insomnia and the attribution process. *Journal of Personality and Social Psychology,* 1970, 16, 319-328.

Stuart, R. B. Behavioral control of overeating. *Behaviour Research and Therapy,* 1967, 5, 357-365.

Stuart, R. B. A three-dimensional program for the treatment of obesity. *Behaviour Research and Therapy,* 1971, 9, 177-186.

Stuart, R. B. Situational versus self-control. In R. D. Rubin, H. Fensterheim, J. D. Henderson, and L. P. Ullman (Eds.), *Advances in Behavior Therapy.* New York: Academic Press, 1972, pp. 129-146.

Stuart, R. B. Behavioral control of overeating: A status report. Paper presented at the Fogarty International Center Conference on Obesity, Bethesda, Maryland, October, 1973.

Stuart, R. B., and Davis, B. *Slim chance in a fat world: Behavioral control of obesity.* Champaign, Ill.: Research Press Co., 1972.

Stunkard, A. J. The dieting depression. *American Journal of Medicine,* 1957, 12, 77-86.

Stunkard, A. J. The management of obesity. *New York State Journal of Medicine,* 1958, 58, 79-87.

Stunkard, A. J. Obesity and the denial of hunger. *Psychosomatic Medicine,* 1959, 21, 281-288.

Stunkard, A. J. New therapies for the eating disorders: Behavior modification of obesity and anorexia nervosa. *Archives of General Psychiatry,* 1972, 26, 391-398.

Stunkard, A. J., and Koch, C. The interpretation of gastric motility: I. Apparent bias in the reports of hunger by obese persons. *Archives of General Psychiatry*, 1964, *11*, 74-82.

Stunkard, A. J., and Mahoney, M. J. Behavioral treatment of the eating disorders. In H. Leitenberg (Ed.), *Handbook of behavior modification*. Englewood Cliffs: Prentice Hall, in press.

Stunkard, A. J. and McLaren-Hume, M. The results of treatment for obesity. *Archives of Internal Medicine*, 1959, *103*, 79-85.

Stunkard, A. J., and Rush, J. Dieting and depression re-examined: A critical review of reports of untoward responses during weight reduction for obesity. *Annals of Internal Medicine*, 1974, *81*, 526-533.

Stutz, R. M., Warm, J. S., and Woods, W. A. Temporal perception in obese and normal-weight subjects: A test of the stimulus-binding hypothesis. *Bulletin of the Psychonomic Society*, 1974, *3*, 23-24.

Swanson, D. W., and Dinello, F. A. Follow up of patients starved for obesity. *Psychosomatic Medicine*, 1970, *32*, 209-214.

Taller, H. *Calories don't count.* New York: Simon and Schuster, 1961.

Task Force on Arteriosclerosis of the National Heart and Lung Institute. *Arteriosclerosis, Volume 1.* Washington, D. C.: United States Department of Health, Education, and Welfare, Public Health Service, DHEW Publication Number (NIH)72-137, 1971.

Terrace, H. S. Stimulus control. In W. K. Honig (Ed.), *Operant behavior: Areas of research and application.* New York: Appleton-Century-Crofts, 1966.

Thomas, D. W., and Mayer, J. Hunting the secret of fat. *Psychology Today*, 1973, *7*, 74-79.

Thoresen, C. E., and Mahoney, M. J. *Behavioral self-control.* New York: Holt, Rinehart & Winston, 1974.

Thorn, G. W. In Wintrobe et al., *Harrison's Principles of Internal Medicine.* New York: McGraw Hill, 1970 (Chap. 48, p. 265).

Thorpe, J. G., Schmidt, E., Brown, P. T., and Castell, D. Aversion-relief therapy: A new method for general application. *Behaviour Research and Therapy*, 1964, *2*, 71-82.

Tullis, F. I. Rational diet construction for mild and grand obesity. *Journal of the American Medical Association*, 1973, *226*, 70-71.

Ullmann, L. P., and Krasner, L. Introduction. In L. P. Ullmann and L. Krasner (Eds.), *Case studies in behavoir modification.* New York: Holt, Rinehart and Winston, 1965, pp. 1-63.

Ullmann, L. P., and Krasner, L. *Case studies in behavior modification.* New York: Holt, Rinehart and Winston, 1965.

Ulrich, R., Stachnik, T., and Mabry, J. *Control of human behavior: From cure to prevention, Vol. 2.* Glenview, Ill.: Scott, Foresman & Co., 1970.

United States Department of Agriculture. *Fatty acids in foods.* Washington, D. C.: United States Department of Agriculture, Home Economics Research Report #7, 1959.

United States Department of Commerce. Statistical Abstract of the United States. Washington, D. C.: U.S. Government Printing Office, 1974.

United States Department of Health, Education, and Welfare. *Facts from FDA,* Publication No. (FDA) 73-2036. Rockville, MD., 1973.

United States Public Law 91-222, Public Health Cigarette Act of 1969. United States Statutes at Large 1970-71. Washington, D. C.: U.S. Government Printing Office, 1971.

Vague, J., and Vague, Ph. Obesity and atherosclerosis. In H. Greten, R. Levine, E. F. Pfeiffer, and A. E. Renold (Eds.), *Lipid metabolism, obesity, and diabetes mellitus: Impact upon atherosclerosis. International symposium, April, 1972.* Stuttgart: George Thieme Publishers, 1974. Pp. 164-168.

Waters, W. F., and McCallum, R. N. The basis of behavior therapy, mentalistic or behavioristic? A reply to E. A. Locke. *Behaviour Research and Therapy,* 1973, *11*, 157-164.

Weininger, J., and Briggs, G. M. Nutrition update, 1974. *Journal of Nutrition Education,* 1974, *6*, 139-143.

Welles, S. L. Nutritive intake of members of weight reduction programs. Unpublished master's thesis, The Pennsylvania State University, 1973.

Werner, S. C. Comparison between weight reduction on a high-calorie, high fat diet and on an isocaloric regimen high in carbohydrate. *New England Journal of Medicine,* 1955, *252*, 661-665.

Westlake, R. J., Levitz, L. S., and Stunkard, A. J. A day hospital program for treating obesity. *Hospital and Community Psychiatry,* 1974, *25*, 609-611.

White, P. Zen macrobiotic diets. *Journal of the American Medical Association,* 1971, *218*, 397.

Wiest, W. M. Some recent criticisms of behaviorism and learning theory. *Psychological Bulletin,* 1967, *67*, 214-225.

Wijesinghe, B. Massed electrical aversion treatment of compulsive eating. *Journal of Behavior Therapy and Experimental Psychiatry,* 1973, *4*, 133-135.

Williams, R. H. *Textbook of endocrinology.* Philadelphia, Pa.: Saunders, 1968.

Wilson, W. S., Hulley, S. B., Burrows, M. I., and Nichaman, Z. Serial lipid and lipoprotein responses to the American Heart Association fat-controlled diets. *American Journal of Medicine,* 1971, *51*, 492-501.

Wollersheim, J. P. Effectiveness of group therapy based upon learning principles in the treatment of overweight women. *Journal of Abnormal Psychology,* 1970, *76*, 462-474.

Wolpe, J. *The practice of behavior therapy.* New York: Pergamon Press, 1969.

Wooley, S. C., Tennenbaum, D., and Wooley, O. W. A naturalistic observation of the influence of palatability on food choices of obese and nonobese. Unpublished manuscript.

Wooley, O. W., and Wooley, S. C. Appetite for palatable food as a function of the caloric density of the previous meal. Paper presented at Eastern Psychological Association, April 19, 1974.

Wooley, O. W., and Wooley, S. C. The experimental psychology of obesity. In T. Silverstone (Ed.), *Obesity: Its pathogenesis and management.* Lancaster: Medical and Technical Publishing Company, 1975.

World Health Organization. Classification of hyperlipidaemias and hyperlipoproteinaemias. *Bulletin of the World Health Organization,* 1970, *43*, 891-916.

Wyden, P. *The overweight society.* New York: William Morrow, 1965.

Yates, A. J. Symptoms and symptom substitution. *Psychological Review,* 1958, *65*, 371-374.

Yates, A. J. *Behavior therapy.* New York: John Wiley, 1970.

Young, C. Planning the low calorie diet. *American Journal of Clinical Nutrition,* 1960, *8*, 896-900.

Young, C. M. Weight control in a college situation. *Postgraduate Medicine,* 1972, *51*, 116-120.

Index

211

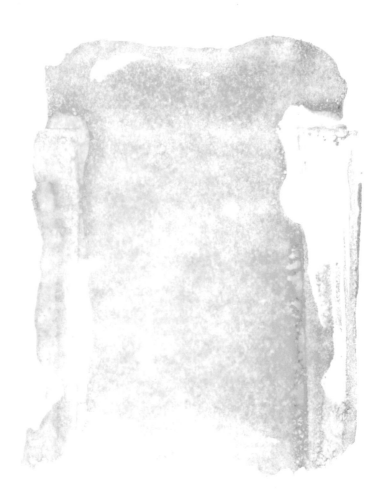